PENGUIN BOOKS

HEART MYTHS

Bruce D. Charash, M.D., is Director of the Cardiac Care Unit at Lenox Hill Hospital in New York and a Fellow of the American College of Cardiology. He lives in New York City with his wife Sarah.

HEART
MYTHS

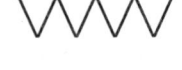

Bruce D. Charash, M.D.

PENGUIN BOOKS

PENGUIN BOOKS
Published by the Penguin Group
Viking Penguin, a division of Penguin Books USA Inc.,
375 Hudson Street, New York, New York 10014, U.S.A.
Penguin Books Ltd, 27 Wrights Lane,
London W8 5TZ, England
Penguin Books Australia Ltd, Ringwood,
Victoria, Australia
Penguin Books Canada Ltd, 10 Alcorn Avenue, Suite 300,
Toronto, Ontario, Canada M4V 3B2
Penguin Books (N.Z.) Ltd, 182–190 Wairau Road,
Auckland 10, New Zealand

Penguin Books Ltd, Registered Offices:
Harmondsworth, Middlesex, England

First published in the United States of America by
Viking Penguin, a division of Penguin Books USA Inc., 1991
Published in Penguin Books 1992

1   3   5   7   9   10   8   6   4   2

A Note to the Reader
The ideas, procedures, and suggestions contained in this book are not intended as a
substitute for consulting with your physician. All matters regarding your health
require medical supervision.

THE LIBRARY OF CONGRESS HAS CATALOGUED THE HARDCOVER AS FOLLOWS:
Charash, Bruce D.
Heart myths/Bruce D. Charash.
p.   cm.
Includes bibliographical references.
ISBN 0-670-82442-9 (hc.)
ISBN 0 14 01.1480 7 (pbk.)
1. Heart—Diseases—Popular works.   2. Medical misconceptions.
I. Title.
RC681.C387   1990
616.1'2—dc20   90–50060

Printed in the United States of America
Set in Bodoni Book
Designed by Ann Gold
Line drawings by Lorraine Walsh

‿‿‿‿‿

Preface

Heart disease is frightening. It is by far the single-biggest killer in the United States, responsible for more than one death every minute. Many of these deaths occur suddenly, without warning, while others occur following heart attacks and bypass surgery. The cost of treating heart disease in this country runs in the tens of billions of dollars annually. The indirect cost is in the hundreds of billions of dollars.

The magnitude of this problem has generated a great deal of public interest. Physicians, the government, and the media have all promoted the public's education. Yet, in spite of this tremendous effort, there remain many *myths* about heart disease and its prevention.

Some of this misinformation is the result of our common desire for simple solutions to complex problems. It is further fueled by the government, through over-generalized health guidelines, and by the media, through sensationalism.

The intention of this book is to explore the most commonly

believed heart myths, and to review the realities and limitations of available scientific information. The topics range from diet to bypass surgery, and from heart murmurs to palpitations. This book is not intended to cover every topic in the field of heart disease, but those which, in my experience, are the most important.

Some of my opinions may be seen as controversial, because they represent an alternative viewpoint. I do not presume to have all of the answers but, instead, wish to point out the limitations of currently held dogma. The truth is often more difficult to accept than the myths themselves. It is my hope that the reader will remain open to all possibilities.

FOR SARAH

I would like to express my gratitude to the following people who provided much appreciated assistance in the preparation of this manuscript: Ruth Knowles, Gerry McCauley, Lorraine Walsh, Dan Frank, Leon Charash, Kathy Robbins, Jeanne Pedersen, and Sarah Charat. And a special thanks to Mary Ann Madden for her invaluable suggestions, and to Michael Millman for his insights, editorial comments, and patience.

VVVVVV

Contents

HEART MYTHS

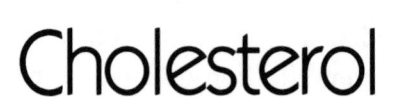

CHAPTER ONE

Cholesterol

Cholesterol is currently a national obsession. Everyone is talking about his or her cholesterol level, and about changing their diets in the hope of preventing heart disease and living longer. But just how much good can we expect by controlling the amount of cholesterol we eat?

Cholesterol was identified as a villain several decades ago when scientists discovered that it accumulated in the walls of arteries, forming blockages. People with higher blood levels of cholesterol were found to be at greater risk for developing heart disease. And nations with higher national cholesterol levels have more heart disease for their population size than nations with lower levels.

It has been established that in the United States the average cholesterol level is relatively high (215 mg/dl)* compared to

---

*"mg/dl" stands for "milligrams per deciliter," which is a measure of the total amount of cholesterol in a small volume of blood.

Japan's (180 mg/dl). More than 25 percent of our adult population have levels greater than 240, and 10 percent have levels greater than 260. Improving diet and lowering the national cholesterol level has become a top-priority public-health issue.

Eat less cholesterol! This message has been spread by doctors, the media, and the food industry. Low-cholesterol food represents a multibillion-dollar-a-year industry. Advertisements more frequently echo the importance of foods that are "cholesterol free" or those that contain oat bran (which may help to lower the blood level of cholesterol although recent scientific evidence has cast doubt on this benefit).

Patients become extremely anxious when they learn that their cholesterol level is elevated. They believe that they must improve their diets (and possibly take cholesterol-lowering medications) in order to prevent premature heart attacks and death.

The U.S. government takes a strong position. It recently criticized American doctors for *not* taking the subject of cholesterol seriously enough. A survey, conducted by the National Heart, Lung, and Blood Institute in 1986, concluded that 50 percent to 75 percent of physicians fail to provide diet or drug treatment for patients with "dangerously" high cholesterol levels. Previously, a panel for the NHLBI recommended that all Americans *over the age of two* adopt a low-fat, low-cholesterol prudent diet.[1]

The government-sponsored panel went even further to suggest that after dietary changes, if one's cholesterol level is still very high (greater than 240), cholesterol-lowering drugs should be considered. The panel judged that doctors are not using these drugs frequently enough.

In effect, the government is recommending a major national effort to change our diets, and in some cases to add medications. This is a far-reaching national health policy. Of course, many of our favorite foods would have to abandoned.

Many people have already made the sacrifice for their health. But others refuse to make changes:

Martin C.,* a fifty-two-year-old accountant with mild heart disease, has a cholesterol level of 280 (which is higher than 95 percent of men his age, and considered dangerously high by the government). He has been advised by his doctor to change his diet. Yet, even knowing that he has heart disease, he refuses to give up steak, butter, and McDonald's. He rarely eats fish and doesn't want to start. "What's the point of living longer if I can't eat what I want?" One doctor prescribed a cholesterol-lowering medication, but it would have cost him more than $150 a month. Martin never filled the prescription.

What benefit can Martin C., as an individual, expect if he changes his diet and takes medications? Will this prevent heart disease? Will he live longer?

There are conflicting and surprisingly disappointing answers to these questions. Yet we have accepted the simplified conclusion that "cholesterol is bad" without full disclosure of the facts. Many people *want* to believe that diet can help them control or prevent heart disease.

Fred E. had a small "warning" heart attack when he was forty-five. He stopped smoking, lost weight, began to exercise, and changed his diet. He gave up most of the foods that were rich in cholesterol and saturated fats. He felt positive about his life.

At fifty-two, he had a second heart attack, and subsequently underwent a triple-bypass operation. Fred became depressed.

*In order to protect their privacy, the names of patients have been fictionalized throughout the book.

"I did everything I was told! What more can I do?" Fred realized that in spite of a successful effort to change his life-style, his heart disease had worsened over the years.

Heart disease cannot always be prevented: a scary and disappointing realization.

Lowering one's cholesterol level may be good, but how good is it? The government, the media, and most doctors never address how realistically *an individual* will benefit by changing his or her diet. What is the promise of these recommendations?

There are many misunderstood facts about cholesterol and many myths of diet. We will explore them.

Myth #1:
Cholesterol is always a bad thing.

We usually think of cholesterol simply as a "villain" responsible for clogging arteries. But most people do not appreciate that cholesterol has a vital biologic function. It is normally produced by the body and used for various purposes. We could not survive without cholesterol in our bodies.

Cholesterol is an integral part of the membrane surrounding every cell in the human body, including the brain. Although we are not sure of its exact role in these membranes, it may help to regulate communication from one cell to another. Cholesterol is also an indispensable chemical "building block," required by the body to make sex hormones, natural steroids, and bile (vital to digestion).

Excessive cholesterol, on the other hand, can certainly be harmful. Cholesterol can deposit in the walls of arteries throughout the body, growing in size over many years to form "plaque" (or atherosclerosis—hardening of the arteries).

The deposits can become so large that they actually block the insides of the arteries, reducing the flow of blood. Blockages in the arteries of the heart can lead to heart attacks and sudden death. Within the circulation to the brain, this can lead to strokes. Extremely excessive cholesterol can also deposit in the skin and tendons, a condition that is usually harmless. It can often be seen during a physical examination as yellow streaks in the skin.

Although too much cholesterol is clearly associated with disease, it is easy to forget how essential it is to our *normal* biologic function.

Myth #2:
There is a normal cholesterol level.

This is not true. There is no simple "normal level." The government would like to see all people with levels below 200. Many laboratories publish a misleading "normal range." In some a level as high as 300 is listed as "normal."

"Normal" is difficult to define. The risk of heart disease is extremely high with a cholesterol level of 330 and is much lower with a level under 180. But the risk is continuous. There is *no* absolutely safe level. However, as seen in the following graph,[2] as the level of cholesterol increases, the risk of heart disease not only increases, but accelerates.

Every incremental increase of 10 brings with it an increasingly greater risk of heart disease.

The average cholesterol level of adults in the United States is approximately 215. More than 25 percent of middle-aged men have levels higher than 240, and over 10 percent have levels higher than 260. Thus, normal is an arbitrary definition.

There are some inherited conditions in which cholesterol

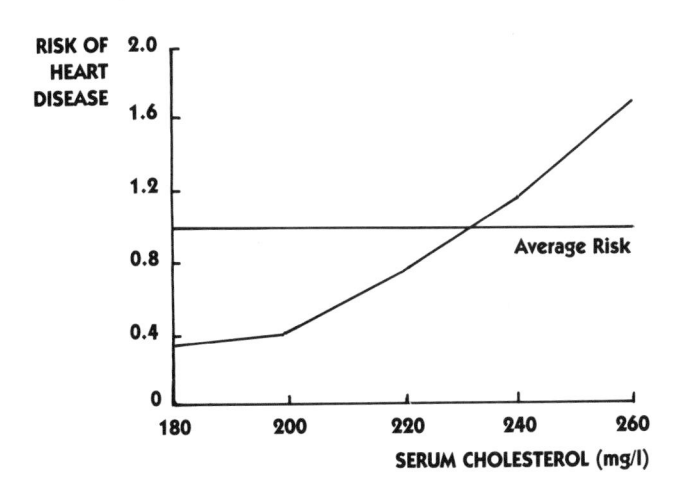

Cholesterol and heart disease in men younger than 50

levels are extremely high (the body is genetically "pro-grammed" to make excessive amounts of cholesterol). The effects are remarkably destructive.

Timmy S. had a heart attack when he was nine years old. His cholesterol level was found to be 980. This level was unchanged by diet. Drugs had almost no effect. He died of a massive heart attack when he was sixteen.

Although this condition (called homozygous familial hy-percholesterolemia) is very rare (only one person in a million has it), it demonstrates the disastrous effect of having a dra-matically high cholesterol level.

Up to 1 in 500 people have a more mild form of this disease (heterozygous familial hypercholesterolemia), in which they have cholesterol levels ranging from 300 to 500. Heart attacks commonly occur when these patients are in their thirties and forties.

Cholesterol Not Important
in Older Men and Women

The risk of heart disease increases with the level of cholesterol in young and middle-aged men and women. But this has *not* been found to be the case in the more elderly patients. According to a large scientific study, those older than sixty years of age with very high cholesterol levels (greater than 260) do *not* have more heart attacks than those with lower cholesterol levels (under 180). A higher level of cholesterol was unrelated to the development of future heart attacks, and death, in these more elderly patients.

The reason for this observation is not fully understood. One theory suggests that people who are vulnerable to the bad effects of cholesterol will have their damage early in life, resulting in heart disease before the age of sixty. If a more elderly person has *not* yet developed heart disease then, the theory continues, he or she may be relatively resistant to the dangerous effects of cholesterol.

With advancing age, high cholesterol levels (greater than 240) become less and less important. It is extremely unlikely that the elderly have much to gain by lowering their cholesterol (since a high level is not important in the first place). This is ironic because older patients are frequently urged by physicians and by the media to change their diets.

Mary N. is almost eighty years old and in good health. She has no evidence of heart disease. Mary refuses to eat butter or red meat. "I'm watching my cholesterol." Her level is 240.

There is no evidence to suggest that Mary needs to watch her cholesterol level, or that lowering it will do her any good. She is a victim of our current cholesterol obsession.

Myth #3:
A low cholesterol level means that
you can't have a heart attack.

This is not true. People have heart attacks even with low cholesterol levels. As stated previously, there is always a risk of heart attacks at any cholesterol level. The risk increases with increasing levels.

Bob Y. is a sixty-four-year-old, previously fit electrician who never smoked cigarettes. He was shocked when he was admitted to the hospital with a heart attack. "My cholesterol level was always low! How could this happen?"

Bob's father had had a heart attack when he was fifty years old. A history of heart disease in the family (especially "early" heart disease) is a major risk factor for heart attacks. Even with a relatively low cholesterol level (Bob's was 170), heart attacks do occur.

Cholesterol can deposit into the lining of arteries for many different reasons, even with low blood levels.

Lou S., a fifty-year-old writer who smoked one pack of cigarettes a day, asked after having a mild heart attack, "What's blocking my arteries? My cholesterol level is low."

The blockages are still made of cholesterol. Cigarette smoking is responsible for accelerating the formation of blockages in this patient.

Why Blockages Develop

Blockages (called atherosclerosis) develop when the cholesterol in our blood deposits inside the lining of our arteries, similar to "sludge" sticking inside a garden hose. But this *sticking* does not occur easily. The artery has a natural protective barrier. The cells that line the inside of the artery resist cholesterol.

Cholesterol must first *seep* through this barrier before it can stick. The process is usually slow. Tiny cholesterol deposits are first seen in the arteries of men and women in their twenties and thirties. It usually takes many more years, even decades, before the blockages grow to be of a clinically important size.

If there is more cholesterol in the blood, there will be more available to seep inside the wall of the artery—a fact dramatically demonstrated by the case of Timmy, the child with a cholesterol level of 980.

With Timmy, the protective barrier was overwhelmed by the huge amount of cholesterol, and deposits grew rapidly inside the arteries of the heart, resulting in a heart attack at age nine.

The level of cholesterol is important in predicting heart disease, but it is not the entire story. Some people will resist high cholesterol levels. They are born with a stronger protective barrier and are less vulnerable to the penetration of cholesterol. Others have congenitally weaker barriers and develop heart disease even with "low" cholesterol levels, not unlike Bob Y., in the example on page 8.

These differences are often hereditary, explaining why some families have a strong history of heart disease (especially in young relatives), while others seem to have very little. Even people born with strong protective barriers in their ar-

9

teries can develop heart disease: the barrier can be made to weaken. An unidentified component of cigarette smoke can cause injury to the protective lining of arteries and "open the door" for cholesterol to enter the arteries and form deposits.

High blood pressure (which pounds on the arteries) and diabetes (a complex disease commonly affecting arteries in the body) can also damage arterial linings. Both of these conditions result in the exaggerated accumulation of cholesterol, and more heart disease.

The development of atherosclerosis is a complex process. A high cholesterol level or excessive injury to the lining of arteries will each contribute to the development of blockages. When an elevated level of cholesterol combines with cigarette smoking, hypertension, or diabetes, the problem is considerably magnified.

On the other hand, in the absence of the previously mentioned conditions (smoking, diabetes, or high blood pressure), a mildly elevated cholesterol level is probably not going to increase significantly the risk of developing heart disease.

We can't control genetic factors. But this does not mean that patients should assume that all is genetic. They will only worsen matters by smoking cigarettes or by not treating high blood pressure. Patients with a strong family history of premature heart disease may be the ones with the most to gain from lowering their cholesterol levels because they are the people at the greatest risk.

Myth #4:
Eating foods with less cholesterol is the most important
way to lower blood cholesterol. Foods that
are cholesterol-free are okay.

This is very commonly misunderstood.

For example, milk is avoided by many heart patients because it contains cholesterol, while most non-dairy coffee whiteners are *cholesterol-free*. This may sound great, but using such products can raise the blood cholesterol level more than by using milk itself.

Only 10 percent to 20 percent of the cholesterol in our blood comes directly from our diet. The majority is manufactured by the liver, the body's cholesterol factory.

If we eat *less* cholesterol, the body makes *more*; and if we eat *more* cholesterol, the body makes *less*. The factory maintains blood cholesterol at a genetically determined level. Those with very high cholesterol levels are programmed to make too much cholesterol in the factory. When these people eat less cholesterol, they only stimulate the factory to make more.

Thus, eating less cholesterol will not by itself do the trick. The most effective way to lower the level of cholesterol is to sabotage the factory by giving it less fuel, thereby preventing the liver from carrying out its mission. It cannot make cholesterol without the proper fuel.

What is this fuel? It is saturated fat.

Saturated fats and oils are converted into cholesterol by the liver. Eating less saturated fat will lessen the production of cholesterol. The most important of these saturated fats include animal fats, coconut oil, and palm oil. In contrast, certain unsaturated fats and fish oils will jam the factory and actually reduce the production of cholesterol.

Many cholesterol-free products (such as the non-dairy coffee whiteners) are rich in palm and coconut oil, and are strong fuels, which raise blood cholesterol levels. Likewise, many health foods such as bran muffins and granola cereals are frequently filled with saturated fats.

Cholesterol is found *only* in animal products. This is also commonly misunderstood—there is no cholesterol in vegetable products. The oils that are used as fuels to make cholesterol, on the other hand, are found in both animal and plant products.

Myth #5:
Some cholesterol is good and some is bad.

We have all heard of good and bad cholesterol. But this is a misconception. All cholesterol is the same. The good/bad difference refers to how cholesterol is packaged as it moves through the blood.

We have described the liver as the cholesterol factory. Cholesterol is taken away *from* the liver in little trucks, called LDL (low-density lipoprotein, which is a combination of fat and protein). These trucks transport cholesterol through the blood to the rest of the body. The cholesterol is released at various sites to be used for both good things: making hormones, building cell membranes; and for what we consider *bad* things: forming deposits in the walls of arteries.

Some cholesterol is rejected by the body and is returned to the factory in a different truck called HDL (high-density lipoprotein). The liver will break this cholesterol back down into little pieces.

Cholesterol carried by HDL, which we call "good" cholesterol, ultimately leaves the body, whereas that carried by LDL is called "bad." There is no difference in the cholesterol

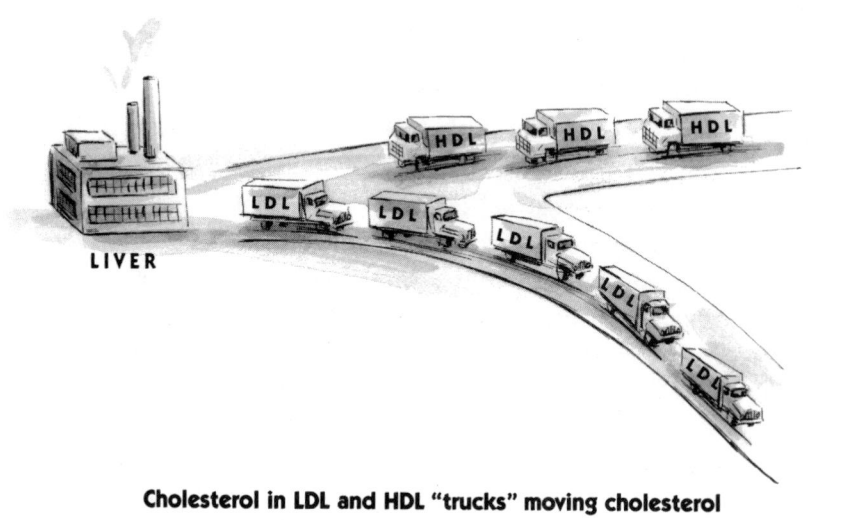

Cholesterol in LDL and HDL "trucks" moving cholesterol

itself, but only in the direction in which it is moving through the body.

There are still several other trucks that carry cholesterol in the blood, but these are found in smaller quantities than either HDL or LDL, and are not important in most people.

When doctors measure total cholesterol in the blood, it includes the cholesterol in all of the trucks. The average person has approximately 80 percent of his or her cholesterol carried by LDL (leaving the liver, and going to the body) and 20 percent by HDL (returning to the liver for destruction). But these percentages can vary.

A person with a total cholesterol level of 260, and 35 percent of it carried by HDL, is better off than another person with the *same total cholesterol level* and only 15 percent of it carried by HDL. The more cholesterol in the HDL form, the more that is being eliminated from the body. The total cholesterol level is not the entire story.

Most laboratories can both measure the total level of cholesterol, *and*, if requested, determine exactly how much of it is carried by LDL and how much is carried by HDL (called "fractionation" of the total cholesterol).

Larry M., a forty-year-old locksmith who smoked one pack of cigarettes a day, suffered a small heart attack. During his recovery, his total cholesterol was measured to be 190 (a relatively low level). However, on fractionation, his HDL cholesterol was discovered to be only 21 (11 percent of the total), an unusually *low* percentage of the total.

Even though Larry's total cholesterol level was not too bad, very little of the cholesterol was found to be leaving his body via the HDL trucks. Although cigarette smoking is the more obvious risk factor, the highly unusual cholesterol metabolism also played an important role in Larry's premature heart disease.

Myth #6:
Lowering your cholesterol has been
shown to make you live longer.

This is the *big myth*.

Although great emphasis has been placed on lowering cholesterol, there is *no* evidence that it will make one live longer. In fact, very few people are aware of what benefits can actually be expected by blood cholesterol reduction. If we as a nation *and as individuals* are to adopt strict government recommendations, we should at least be informed as to the known benefits to be derived.

Consider again Martin C., the fifty-two-year-old accountant mentioned on page 3, with the cholesterol level of 280 mg/dl. Martin does *not* smoke cigarettes, and he has normal blood pressure and *no* diabetes. His doctor has recommended diet, and Martin has refused to consider it. Additionally, Martin will *not* take medications. Is he wrong?

Is Martin placing his life in jeopardy? Will Martin certainly die prematurely if he ignores his doctor's recommendations?

It is well established that men and women younger than 60 years of age with higher cholesterol levels are more likely to develop heart disease. But it is *not* so obvious that *lowering* cholesterol will reduce this risk (especially in the more elderly, in whom cholesterol levels are not related to the development of heart disease).

During the past thirty years, numerous scientific studies have examined this important question, by attempting to lower blood cholesterol through dietary manipulation or the use of medications. However, most of these studies were inconclusive because of their small size or poor study design.

In 1984 a breakthrough occurred. A U.S. government–sponsored study was published, offering the most important results of its time.[3] This study, the Lipid Research Clinic's Coronary Primary Prevention Trial, is extensively quoted by many doctors, scientists, and the media. More than any other study it was used to justify the government's strict dietary recommendations.

Instead of simply accepting that we should *all* modify our diets and lower our cholesterol levels, let us examine the actual information used by the government to form its recommendation.

The LRC-CPPT administered to middle-aged men between thirty-four and fifty years of age with high cholesterol levels, a drug called cholestyramine (which prevents the absorption of cholesterol from the intestines); 3,806 men, with an average cholesterol level of 290, were recruited.

After several months of a cholesterol-lowering diet (ample time to determine a benefit), the average cholesterol level decreased only 10 points, down to 280 (a 4 percent drop, which is less impressive than many had expected).

At this point 1,906 men (approximately half) were given the drug cholestyramine and 1,900 were given a placebo (an inactive substitute that looked just like the real medicine). Neither the doctors nor the patients knew who got the bona fide drug. This information was kept a secret until the end of the study.

The cholestyramine was given to the study's participants free of charge, whereas actual patient costs are as much as $100 a month. Since they are consumers, these patients have the right to know what they are paying for. The results of the study help to answer these questions:

LRC–CPPT

	PLACEBO	DRUG
number of men	1,900	1,906
initial cholesterol (on diet)	280	280
cholesterol after 7 years	277	257
% decrease in cholesterol level	1%	8.5%

After seven years, the average cholesterol level of the placebo group fell by 3 points, whereas the drug group had a more impressive 23-point reduction in their cholesterol level. But the *big question* is: did this 23-point fall in cholesterol improve the health of the men in the study?

These men had much to gain by lowering their cholesterol

levels. Their initial levels were extremely high. Even *after* dieting the average level for the group was higher than 95 percent of all American men. And the men were all younger than fifty years of age (cholesterol levels are more important in younger patients). Therefore, a decrease in the level of cholesterol would be expected to have a big impact.

The men in this study were free of heart disease at the start. The aim was to see if the men taking the drug developed fewer heart problems than those taking the placebo.

LRC–CPPT

	PLACEBO	DRUG
number of men	1,900	1,906
number of men with heart attacks	187	155

During the seven years of the study, there were 187 heart attacks among the 1,900 men on placebo. The same number of heart attacks would have been expected to occur among the men taking cholestyramine. But this group had only 155! This is 32 fewer than expected. Taking the drug therefore prevented 32 men from having heart attacks, a statistically significant reduction for the group.

But 1,906 men had to be treated for seven years to protect these 32 men (who represented only 1.7 percent of all those taking the drug). The majority of men who were treated received no obvious benefit.

The *group* had statistically fewer heart attacks. This may be an important benefit for society. But the individual benefit is very different. An individual has, at best, only a small chance that drugs and diet will prevent heart disease during seven years. And this is for those with the most to gain (young men with

the highest cholesterol levels). Older men with lower cholesterol levels would be expected to receive even less of a benefit.

Deaths Unchanged

Although there were fewer heart attacks among the men taking
the cholestyramine, total death was *unchanged* in the study!

LRC–CPPT

	PLACEBO	DRUG
number of men	1,900	1,906
total number of deaths	71	68
cause of death:		
heart attack	44	32
cancer	15	16
accidents and violence	4	11
other	8	9

As shown in the preceding chart, 71 men died taking the
placebo and 68 men died taking cholestyramine during the
seven years of the study. This is not a statistically significant
difference. Men taking the drug *did not* live longer. Deaths
due to heart attack were definitely reduced. But *non*–heart
attack deaths were increased by nearly an equal amount.

It is exciting that by lowering cholesterol we can reduce
death due to heart disease. But by doing so we observe a
slight increase in the amount of non–heart attack death, thus
offsetting the advantage. As a nation we are all being encouraged to lower our cholesterol levels. *But this policy might
not affect mortality.*

Interestingly, the number of deaths due to accidents and
violence was increased in the group of men taking cholestyra-

mine. The placebo group had only 4 such deaths. The drug group had 11. Although at first this may not seem like a large difference, when compared to heart disease, violent death is not very common in the United States. An increase from 4 to 11 out of roughly 2,000 men (more than doubling the amount) is curious, and possibly more than a random difference.

The violent deaths resulted from a mixture of suicide, homicide, and automobile accidents (some of which were related to alcohol). The scientists who published the study concluded: ". . . since no plausible connection could be established between cholestyramine treatment and violent or accidental death, it is difficult to conclude that this could be anything but a chance occurrence." But is this implausible? Cholesterol is the essential ingredient used to make all sex hormones and naturally occurring steroids. It is also a vital part of all cell membranes, including the cells of the brain. Could the *lowering* of our body level of cholesterol alter our delicate hormonal balance and even affect our personalities and behavior? Is there an interaction with alcohol (which contributed to some of the deaths)?

These issues were *not* considered by the investigators. In retrospect, it would have been interesting to know the levels of certain hormones in the men taking both the placebo and the drug. It would also have been valuable to collect statistics on the personality traits and mood of the study's participants. But this was not done.

The members of the drug group experienced a *reduction* in their cholesterol levels by the end of the study, distinguishing them from the men who are naturally at this lower level. The process of cholesterol reduction makes them different. We will explore this point in more detail later on.

What can we conclude from the study? There are several points to be made:

1. Lowering cholesterol produced a reduction in heart disease (but only in middle-aged men with very high cholesterol levels).

2. Only 1.7 percent of men received a benefit by taking the drug. The majority of men experienced *no* change in outcome. They took the drug and got nothing in return.

3. The chance of dying was *not* changed by taking the medication.

4. Although heart-attack death was less common among the men taking the drug, there was an increase in violent and accidental deaths in this group.

5. The investigators stated that the increase in violent deaths could only be a chance occurrence. But this is only their opinion. It is *not* inconceivable that this difference reflects a real problem with cholesterol reduction. The effect of lowered cholesterol on mood and behavior is unknown.

The government has urged that all people over the age of two adopt the American Heart Association's "Prudent Diet" in an effort to reduce our national cholesterol level. It has further stated that each of us should have our cholesterol level measured. If it is greater than 240, an even more strict diet is advised. If, after diet, it is still greater than 240, cholesterol-reducing medications are to be considered.

But, based on the government's own study, making these changes is unlikely to be of much help. Less than 2 percent of relatively young men with the highest cholesterol levels had been spared a heart attack by aggressive drug therapy. And as we stated before, the number of total deaths was unchanged.

Even less of a benefit would be expected by lowering cholesterol in those with levels under 240. For those with a level between 200 and 240, there are absolutely no data to suggest that anything will be gained by cholesterol reduction.

In 1987 a study from Europe, called the Helsinki Heart Trial, examined the same issues as the American trial.[4] Four thousand middle-aged men with an average cholesterol level of 269 were examined. This time a different drug, called gemfibrozil, was tested on half. This drug helps the blood eliminate cholesterol. A placebo pill was given to the other half.

HELSINKI HEART TRIAL

	PLACEBO	DRUG
number of men	2,030	2,051
initial cholesterol	269	269
cholesterol after 5 years	272	246
% decrease in cholesterol	0%	8%
number of men with heart attacks	84	56

After five years of follow-up, the men taking the drug had a 23 point fall in their level of cholesterol. Those taking the placebo, in contrast, had a small and insignificant increase in their level.

As in the American LRC-CPPT, there was a significant reduction in cardiac events among the men taking the drug. There were 84 heart attacks in the placebo group and only 56 in the gemfibrozil group, a statistically significant reduction for the group. But once again the individual's benefit was *not* impressive. The drug group of more than two thousand had 28 fewer heart attacks than expected, representing only 1.4 percent of the men who were treated. This is amazingly similar to the result of the LRC-CPPT study. One hundred men had to be treated for five years to prevent fewer than two heart attacks. Again, the majority of the men took the drug and received *no* benefit!

Equally remarkable is that this study also *failed* to demonstrate a difference in death.

HELSINKI HEART TRIAL

	PLACEBO	DRUG
number of men	2,030	2,051
total number of deaths	42	45
cause of death:		
heart attack	19	14
cancer	11	11
accidents and violence	4	10
other	8	10

Both groups had roughly the same number of men die. Death from heart attack was slightly reduced by the drug but non-heart-related death was likewise increased. And, as in the cholestyramine study, there was an increase (more than a doubling) in *violent and accidental deaths* among the men taking the drug.

The Helsinki Heart publication states: "An excess number of violent deaths in subjects treated with lipid-lowering regimens has also been observed in other studies, but has been interpreted to be a chance finding."

Two major studies conducted in two different countries, using two different drugs, have both found an increase in violent/accidental deaths among men experiencing a reduction in their cholesterol levels. Even though the actual numbers are not very large, this is a disturbing finding. It is equally disturbing that this fact has been virtually disregarded by the studies' investigators. It may be a random finding, coincidental to both studies. But it may also be a subtle, and real, difference. We do not know.

No difference in cancer rates was found in either study. In the past, lower cholesterol levels have been associated with increased cancer risk. This caused concern among the investigators, who were relieved to find no difference in the rate of cancer between the drug and placebo groups. However, the two studies followed men for only seven and five years, respectively. Cancer takes more time to develop. The long-term effects of cholesterol reduction are still unknown. We cannot predict the incidence of cancer after, let us say, twenty years of cholesterol reduction. A difference might be found with the passage of more time.

Interestingly, in the late 1970s a different drug study was published, with very disturbing results.[5] The drug tested, clofibrate, reduced cholesterol levels, resulting in a reduction in the amount of heart disease. And, as in the cholestyramine and gemfibrozil studies, the individual benefit was seen in only 1.5 percent of men taking the drug.

But in this study total death was *significantly increased* among the men taking the drug (from 127 out of 5,000 men on placebo, to 162 out of 5,000 men on clofibrate). The drug itself was responsible for the increased death rate, because it had a serious effect on the liver, gallbladder, and intestines. This study serves as an important reminder that there are risks involved when administering all drugs (although this was a most dramatic example). Although clofibrate reduced the chance of dying from a heart attack, it increased the overall chance of death. The drug is still available on the market, but is prescribed only with caution.

In summary, it is now accepted that lowering cholesterol will reduce the chance of developing heart disease. The two major trials have demonstrated that groups of middle-aged men who start with very high cholesterol levels will have an impressive statistical reduction in heart disease if they take cholesterol-lowering medications. But each *individual* treated will have less than a 2 percent likelihood of benefiting from therapy (during a five- to seven-year period of time). And the chance of dying will not change.

There are very few examples of individuals or populations *living longer* because they have low cholesterol levels. For example, Greenland has a very low national cholesterol level, attributed to the public's great consumption of fish, and likewise has a low annual death rate from heart disease. Yet the average life expectancy of men in Greenland is 59.7 years, while in the United States it is 71.2 years. Although Greenland's population has lower cholesterol levels and less heart disease, people *do not* live longer as a result.

Yet the U.S. government adheres to its recommendation that all Americans over the age of two should be on a cholesterol- and fat-reduced diet. The American Heart Association has supported this policy, urging the use of their "Prudent Diet."[6] However, not all scientists have agreed with this recommendation.

The consensus panel of fourteen scientists who published the original government report had some dissent among its members. Additionally, the American Academy of Pediatrics has voiced concern that the *safety* of this diet has not been established in growing children.[7] In fact, there have been some reports of children suffering from stunted growth and malnutrition because parents placed them on diets that were too strict.

The Food and Nutrition Board of the National Academy of Science has stated that most people do not need to worry about lipid modification.[8] Even the American Medical Association has stated that a more individualized approach to cholesterol reduction may be more appropriate.[9] The AMA emphasized that men in the upper ninetieth percentile of cholesterol levels are the ones who need the most attention. (The government recommends more aggressive dietary changes for men within the upper twenty-fifth percentile).

Numerous papers in the scientific community have made reference to cholesterol hysteria in the United States. Yet, in spite of the facts and the criticism by many scientists and organizations, most Americans have simply accepted the evils of eating cholesterol.

Most people (especially those with known heart disease) want to believe that they can have some control over their illness. They want to believe that diet can protect them. But the facts speak for themselves. Most individuals will derive absolutely no benefit from cholesterol reduction. One scientist predicted that if an average person, without major risk factors from heart disease, were to use diet modification and lower his cholesterol by 7 percent he would *at best* expect to extend his life expectancy by three days to three months. But even this is conjecture. No one has demonstrated that life expectancy will improve through cholesterol reduction.

Many people do not want to face these facts. I inform my patients that aggressive dietary changes may lead only to a 3 percent to 10 percent reduction in blood cholesterol. Even if their cholesterol level is very high (greater than 260), I tell them that the impact of dietary changes may be very small. They may have only a 1 percent to 2 percent chance of avoiding a heart attack by lowering cholesterol. And there is no evidence that they will live longer.

Further, if they are older than sixty years of age, there may be absolutely no effect by changing their diet. It their cho-lesterol level is lower than 240 at any age, there is no data to suggest that diet will help either.

However, if some of my patients have very high cholesterol levels (greater than 300), or if they have other significant cardiac risk factors (smoking, hypertension, or diabetes), then the risk of developing heart disease is dramatically increased. It is unproven, but more likely, that these people might benefit from aggressive cholesterol reduction.

Diet modification and drug therapy are reasonable courses if used with clinical perspective. But we have lost that per-spective. Medicine cannot be practiced by wish fulfillment. The available data suggest that moderation may be the best approach. More aggressive and indiscriminate therapy is not justified.

∧∧∧∧∧

CHAPTER TWO

Hypertension

Hypertension (high blood pressure) affects up to 40 million Americans. In the United States it is the most common reason people see doctors, and the most common reason people fill prescriptions at drugstores. There has been a strong national drive to make people aware of their blood pressure. Screening occurs not only at the doctor's office, but at work, health fairs, and shopping centers. As a result, it is estimated that 75 percent of adults have had their blood pressure measured.

Yet, in spite of this effort, hypertension remains one of the most misunderstood of medical illnesses. Most people have only a vague idea of what it is or why we treat it. Some people think that hypertension has something to do with people who are "hyper" (excitable, type-A personalities). This is a common *myth*. There are many other myths and misconceptions concerning hypertension. Among them is the myth that everyone with hypertension *absolutely must* be treated. This is not true.

The use of salt is also misunderstood. There has been a major effort to encourage all of us to reduce the amount of salt in our diets (salt is commonly linked to high blood pressure). But there is no reason why *everyone* must avoid salt. This is a greatly exaggerated health concern.

To help us understand hypertension, let's look at a typical example:

> Ron G. is a forty-four-year-old man who works as a computer programmer. He has "mild" hypertension, with a blood pressure of 145/94 recorded during his last visit with the doctor. He is otherwise healthy, and does *not* smoke cigarettes. His cholesterol is 185 (considered desirable by the government). His blood pressure was *not* improved by giving up salt, so his doctor added a diuretic (more commonly known as a water pill). However, his blood pressure remained elevated. His doctor then added a drug called propranolol, which is a member of the group of medications called beta-blocker.
>
> The treatment succeeded in lowering Ron's blood pressure to 135/85. But Ron began to complain of feeling weak at work. He also started to have some sexual dysfunction and was afraid that he was becoming impotent. His doctor said they would consider switching drugs if the symptoms persisted, but reminded Ron, "We must control your blood pressure. You don't want to die of a stroke, do you?" Ron agreed that he would continue to take medicines to control his hypertension.

Ron is typical of many Americans with hypertension. He has mild disease—his blood pressure is only mildly elevated. Of the 40 million people in the United States estimated to have hypertension, 70 percent are considered to have mild cases. The remaining 30 percent have moderate to severe disease, with more elevated blood pressure readings.

The decision to treat Ron with drugs—giving a water pill

first and then adding a beta-blocker, like propranolol—is considered standard care by many physicians in this country. However, this *standard* approach to hypertension is obsolete, over-aggressive, and flawed!

Ron has been persuaded that he will live longer if he takes drugs. But he may be misled about the benefits of drug therapy. As a consumer of health care, he is entitled to know how likely he *as an individual* will benefit from therapy. Will he really live longer? Will he be more healthy? Does he have to take drugs?

Drugs are overused in this country. They are often expensive and have multiple side effects. In fact, the aggressive use of diuretics has, in some scientific studies, been found to backfire and *increase* the amount of death among some people with mild hypertension. Consequently, when we use drugs we should be sure that the benefits outweigh the risks. But this is not always the case. We may be using the wrong drugs in many people.

We will now explain some of the basics of hypertension and salt and dispel some basic myths and misunderstandings. Then we will turn to the complex issue of whether drugs are needed for all people.

What Is High Blood Pressure?

Blood travels through our body in tubes called arteries (or blood vessels). These vessels are constantly under pressure as the blood moves through them. The heart's pumping action drives the blood forward, creating pressure. Each heartbeat pushes the pressure in the arteries upward. The pressure reaches a peak, and then it drifts back down to a minimum level. The next heartbeat pushes the pressure up once again.

The highest pressure in the arteries, achieved at the peak

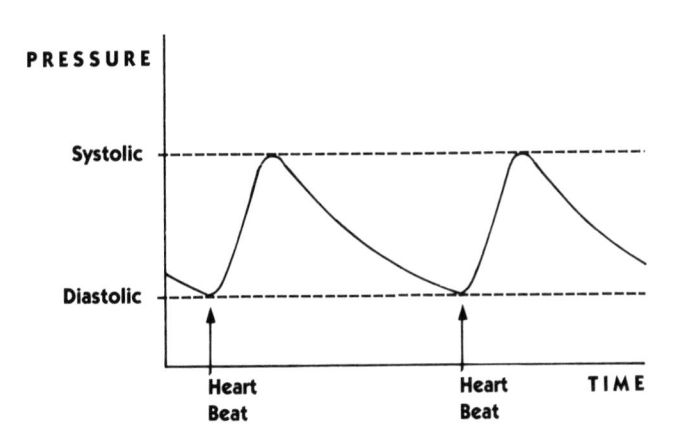

PRESSURE

Systolic

Diastolic

Heart
Beat

Heart
Beat

TIME

Blood pressure during each heartbeat

of the heart's pumping, is called the systolic pressure. For Ron G., in the previous example, it was 145 mm Hg (millimeters of mercury). The lowest pressure (just before the next heartbeat) is called the diastolic pressure. In Ron, it was 94 mm Hg. As a result, we described Ron's blood pressure as 145/94 (in medical parlance, "145 over 94").

As total blood pressure increases, both the upper (systolic) and lower (diastolic) numbers can increase. However, the diastolic number is considered the more important. It is the pressure in the arteries when the heart is the most relaxed. Many things can temporarily drive the systolic (peak) pressure upward. But when the lowest number is elevated there is more likely to be a real problem with the circulation of blood. Increased diastolic numbers indicate that even when the heart is relaxed the pressure in the blood vessels is too high.

We usually say that in adults the systolic pressure (peak pressure) should be under 160. The diastolic pressure (the lower number, and the more important one) should be under 90.

Myth #1:
There is such a thing as normal blood pressure.

This is not true. "Normal" has been arbitrarily defined. But there is no absolutely safe value of blood pressure. The risk of developing heart disease or having a stroke increases with increasing blood pressure. This is especially true when the diastolic value increases over 104. But complications can develop in people with lower readings.

Hypertension has been divided into different categories based on the diastolic number as follows:

DIASTOLIC READING

Normal	less than 89
Mild	90–104
Moderate	105–114
Severe	greater than 115

We have defined under 90 as "normal" for the diastolic pressure. Yet people with "normal" diastolic values between 80 and 90 have double the chance of developing heart disease than those with values between 60 and 70 (which also falls in this same broad "normal" category). The risk is relatively low for both groups, but it is better to have a lower value of blood pressure. *There is no absolutely safe level.* People with the lowest values can still die of strokes and heart attacks.

As we mentioned earlier, 70 percent of all people with

hypertension have mild disease, with diastolic readings between 90 and 104. The remaining 30 percent have a diastolic reading above 104, in the moderate and severe categories.

Blood pressure is a measure of the "wear and tear" of the blood vessels in the body. Higher blood pressure means there is greater pounding of blood as it passes through the arteries. This can result in damage to the arteries, allowing cholesterol to stick more easily to their walls. But this damage does *not* occur in all people with hypertension, because some tolerate the pounding better than others.

The damage is greater in people who have other risk factors for heart disease. This is especially true in smokers and those with elevated cholesterol and/or diabetes. The role of hypertension becomes increasingly important in these people, in part because these other conditions also lead to the damage of blood vessels. When they are mixed with hypertension, the damage is multiplied.

By the same token an elevated blood pressure is of less concern in the absence of these other conditions. Hence it may *not* be so urgent to treat it. In the case on page 28, Ron G. had mild hypertension, without other cardiac risk factors. It is *not* clear that drug therapy was indicated; it could at least have been delayed while exploring non-drug therapy.

Myth #2:
People who are "hyper" are people with hypertension.

People frequently assume that *only* aggressive, agitated people have high blood pressure. This is not true. Blood pressure is often elevated in people who are relaxed and calm, and many "hyper" people have normal blood pressure.

Hypertension is a complex condition involving a combination of excessive fluid in the body's circulation, and increased squeezing of the muscles surrounding the arteries (which carry blood from the heart). It is *not* a simple reflection of personality.

Although becoming upset will raise blood pressure temporarily in most of us, this is *not* what causes chronic hypertension. Because most people are anxious about going to their doctor, their blood pressure can be 10 to 15 mm Hg higher in the doctor's office. This has been confirmed by tests using special blood pressure cuffs that take measurements automatically at home. As a result, elevated blood pressure in the doctor's office does not always mean that the patient has hypertension. Repeat measurements after the patient relaxes, and after repeated office visits, may reveal a normal blood pressure.

Myth #3:
"I can sense when my blood pressure is high."

This is another common, and occasionally dangerous, *myth*. Certain symptoms are frequently associated with hypertension, such as headache, nosebleed, dizziness, and fainting. Although people with hypertension often report these symptoms to their doctors, they are found *as frequently* in people with normal blood pressure. In addition, the presence of these symptoms does not correspond to the periods of time when blood pressure is the highest in those with hypertension.

Many people *assume* that if they do not have a headache, then their blood pressure is acceptable. This can be dangerously misleading. Symptoms are *not* a barometer of blood pressure. Hypertension is truly a "silent" disease in most people.

James S., a fifty-three-year-old man who was on a "pressure pill" for years, was uncomfortable with the side effects of the medication. Yet, as with most people, the high blood pressure never had caused any symptoms. On his own, James decided abruptly to stop his pills. He felt well and had no complaints. He never experienced a headache.

Four days later his wife found him unresponsive in a chair, where he had been reading a book. James had suffered a major stroke and died later that day. Abruptly stopping his pills caused a surge in his blood pressure, and this proved to be lethal. Although his blood pressure was extremely elevated, James had no warning symptoms.

Hypertension can indeed cause some of the side effects mentioned previously. But most people will feel nothing when their pressure is very elevated. A stroke can be the first symptom.

Unfortunately, the drugs we use for hypertension have plenty of potential side effects. These include impotence, headache, weakness, depression, dizziness, dry mouth, rash, constipation, insomnia, and nausea. It can also be very dangerous to stop taking blood pressure pills abruptly once they have been started. The sudden discontinuation of many pills can induce a "rebound" effect in which the blood pressure can shoot up to higher values than before the drug was started, and, as in the case of James, can lead to stroke and death. *Most medications should therefore be discontinued only under medical supervision.*

It is certainly possible that physicians make some people *feel worse* by treating their high blood pressure with drugs. The purpose of therapy, however, is not to make people feel better day to day, but to avoid the terrible long-term complications of high blood pressure. But, besides the actual dollar expense of drugs, there is a cost in side effects for many people. Although most people can eventually have their blood pressure controlled by taking drugs that they tolerate, some can not. What is the individual benefit of taking pills for high blood pressure? We will explore this point later in the chapter.

Myth #4:
Hypertension is the same disease in all people who have it.

Blood pressure is nothing more than a physical measurement of the pressure in a given person's circulation. Pressure in the circulation can be elevated above what we define as "normal" for many different reasons. Elevated pressure is called hypertension, regardless of the reason. It is not in itself a disease but rather a reflection of one of many different underlying conditions.

Poor blood circulation to the kidneys, certain tumors, and some malformations of the circulation can all cause blood pressure to be elevated. The resultant hypertension is called "secondary." It is secondary to the underlying condition. However, secondary hypertension is found in only a very small number of people, because these collective conditions are very uncommon.

The majority of people with hypertension do *not* have an identifiable underlying cause. These cases are called "primary" or "essential" hypertension, which we have lumped together as if it were one disease. But this simple label merely reflects our inability to understand the hypertension.

Is it logical to assume that nearly 40 million people with essential hypertension all suffer from the *same disease?* Although we do not *yet* know how to identify and measure all the different mechanisms of essential hypertension, we have made remarkable advances in our understanding of these differences. We have recently begun to understand that essential hypertension is *not* a single disease.

This is not a trivial distinction. Consider fever. Fever is not itself a disease. Rather, it is an elevation of the body temperature, which can be the result of many different underlying diseases and conditions. Not all fevers will require treatment, as in a minor viral cold, whereas more serious bacterial infections may require the administration of intravenous antibiotics. Aspirin and Tylenol can lower the temperature and make people feel better, but this course of treatment is not always required.

Obviously, when we diagnose a fever we first define the underlying cause. Then we direct proper therapy (if therapy is needed at all). Using one drug for everybody, or only one approach to treating all fever, would be inappropriate.

Similarly, hypertension is not one disease and cannot be approached in a single way. But for years we employed one approach to treating all patients with essential hypertension: "stepped care." As seen in the example of Ron on page 28, the first step is for *all* patients with high blood pressure to consume less salt. The next step is to add a water pill. And if this is not effective, a beta-blocking drug (such as propranolol) is introduced. Finally, other drugs are added if needed. This stepped care approach has been used for years by most physicians in the United States.

But our state of knowledge has taught us that stepped care is no longer a proper way to treat this problem. In fact, not all patients with hypertension require therapy. Additionally, not all patients with hypertension need to avoid salt.

Some may even do *worse* with salt restriction. And many patients should *not* be on a water pill. We can best understand the different mechanisms of hypertension by exploring the role of salt and its effect on blood pressure. We will divide hypertension into two groups: "volume" hypertension and "squeezing" hypertension.

Myth #5:
Everyone should avoid salt. Certainly all people with high blood pressure must *avoid salt.*

This is an exaggerated health concern that has invaded every household in the advertising of innumerable "salt free" (and often taste-free) products. We are constantly reminded to consume less salt, and are often subjected to criticism if we pick up a salt shaker. Yet *most* people do not have to avoid salt, including many with hypertension.

With all the public "salt" awareness, most of us do not know why salt is considered harmful or why it has such a bad reputation. What does extra salt do to the body?

Salt and the Body

We need salt to live. It is a vital part of all body fluids. The salt we eat eventually enters the bloodstream. It pulls water by osmosis into the circulation with it. The more salt we eat, the more water is pulled into the blood system.

Eating excessive salt (more than is needed by the body) pulls with it excessive water, which expands the volume of blood. This causes the pressure to increase inside the circulation, just as adding extra water into a filled water balloon exerts increased pressure on the balloon's walls.

When blood pressure is elevated because of the extra salt and water, we call it "volume" hypertension. Patients with this form of hypertension will lower their pressure by avoiding salt and by taking water pills. Both approaches treat the

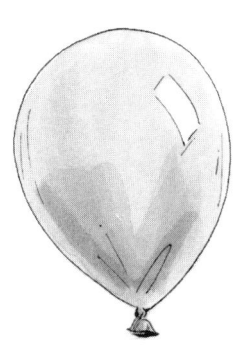 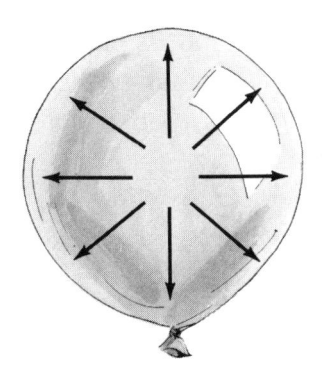

Adding more water increases the balloon's internal pressure.

underlying volume problem. However, many people with hypertension (up to 20 percent) are completely *unaffected* by salt.

These people do *not* have a volume problem. Instead, they have high blood pressure because the arteries in their body are being squeezed from the outside. We could make the analogy of a hand squeezing our water balloon from the outside: the volume of fluid inside the balloon is normal, but the pressure is increased because the walls are squeezed into the fluid.

A layer of muscle surrounds every artery in the body. Each layer has the potential to squeeze down (called vasoconstriction). When this occurs, blood pressure increases. The more squeezing there is, the greater the increase of blood pressure, which we call "squeezing" hypertension (more technically, vasoconstrictive hypertension).

A hormone made in the kidneys called renin causes these muscles to "squeeze." The more renin released from the kidneys, the more the blood vessels constrict, and the greater the increase in blood pressure. Squeezing hypertension is caused by too much renin.

Medicines are available that can relax the muscles that surround the arteries of the body. These drugs effectively

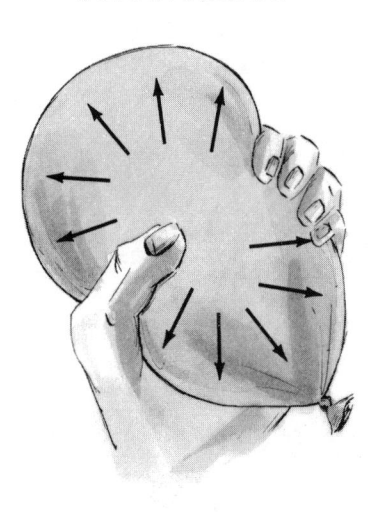

Squeezing the balloon increases internal pressure.

lower the blood pressure in those with squeezing hypertension. Avoiding salt, on the other hand, will not work since these people do not have a problem with extra volume.

Avoiding salt can even worsen matters for people with squeezing hypertension. The kidneys overreact to the shrinking volume of blood by releasing greater and greater amounts of renin. This leads to more and more squeezing on the arteries. As the blood volume gets smaller, the squeezing gets greater. The net effect on blood pressure might be that it would stay the same, or even increase.

The following graph demonstrates the change in blood pressure induced by avoiding salt in people with the volume-type hypertension, who have too much salt and water in their circulation.[1] It is very impressive. However, people with the squeezing type of blood pressure do not have an impressive change. In fact, the diastolic reading actually increased for the group.

Avoiding salt can potentially harm people with squeezing

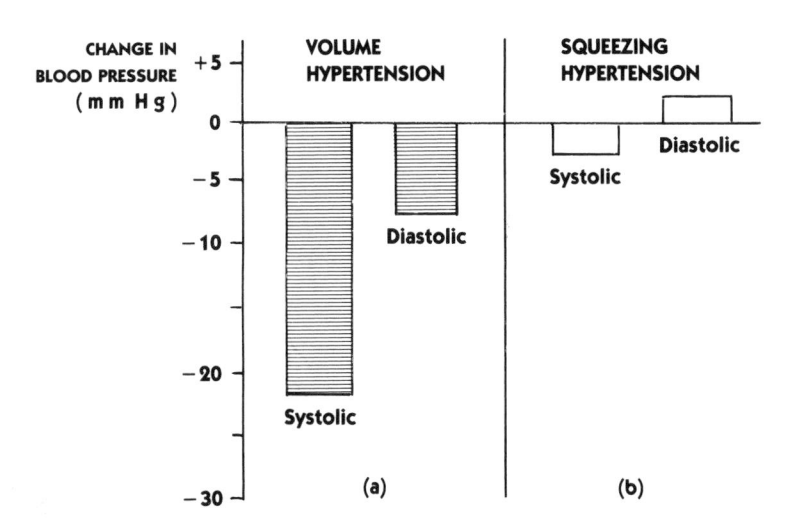

How Avoiding Salt Affects Blood Pressure

Patients with volume hypertension (a) experience a large fall in their systolic and diastolic pressures; patients with squeezing hypertension (b) reveal little change with salt reduction.

hypertension. Besides risking a slight increase in blood pressure , there is a further danger related to the greater muscular squeezing provoked by the avoidance of salt in these patients.

Elevated blood pressure results in damage to arteries (in both the volume and squeezing groups) because of the increased pounding. However, the squeezing group has *extra* damage because the constriction of the surrounding muscles further traumatizes the arteries, thus worsening the situation. It has been observed that patients with squeezing hypertension have more heart attacks and strokes than those with volume hypertension.

Thus, by avoiding salt, those people with squeezing hypertension will experience even more renin release and a greater amount of external squeezing. This is harmful in the long run. These patients may be better off eating as much salt as they want. Eating extra salt can turn down the renin level and lead to relaxation of blood vessels.

Therefore, we can divide hypertension into different categories: 1. squeezing hypertension (20 percent): caused by high levels of the hormone renin, and having normal amounts of salt/water in the blood; 2. volume hypertension (30 percent): caused by excessive salt/water, and low levels of the hormone renin; and 3. mixed squeezing/volume (50 percent): caused by a mixture of moderately elevated renin levels, and moderately excessive salt/water.

How Can You Tell Which Type of High Blood Pressure You Have?

Renin levels can be measured in people with high blood pressure. If the renin level is very high, then we conclude that the blood pressure is elevated because of the squeezing on the arteries. We treat these patients with drugs that relax the muscles, and actually encourage these people *not* to avoid salt.

If the renin level is low, then the problem is related to extra volume. These people will benefit from avoiding salt (to reduce the volume of blood.) They also respond to diuretics (water pills). If the renin level is normal, we conclude that the high blood pressure is of the mixed volume/squeezing form and the response to salt reduction and the various medications is likewise mixed.

Diuretics

There are many types of diuretics on the market. These medicines all work by interfering with the normal function of the kidneys, forcing them to spill extra salt and water into the urine. They can *all* be harmful to the kidneys, especially if very large doses are administered.

Those with too much salt and water in the their body (volume-hypertensive, with low renin levels) will respond most effectively to water pills. For people with the squeezing type of hypertension, these pills will do little good. The mixed group will have a mixed response.

In the example on page 28, Ron was given one of these pills. His blood pressure had no response, indicating that he might be in the squeezing group. The diuretic was ineffective, yet his doctor left him on that medicine (as part of the standard stepped care approach). However, Ron was being exposed only to the potential harm of the diuretics, without receiving any benefit.

Diuretics have many bad side effects. They can increase cholesterol levels in the blood, they can worsen diabetes, and there is a small chance that they can cause impotence. The most significant side effect is to lower the blood level of potassium (an important mineral in the body's electrical balance.)

Potassium is found in all bodily fluids. It is vital to many bodily functions, including the regulation of the electricity of the heart. Most diuretics will cause potassium to be wasted in the urine, along with the salt.

If the level of potassium gets too low, the heart can have dangerous (and potentially fatal) changes of its electrical rhythm. In fact, one major scientific study found that sudden death was *more common* in people who were given extra diuretics (about twice the dose we usually use) for their hypertension. We learned that for diuretics "less is more."

Although most people on diuretics are also given potassium pills, these pills rarely keep pace with the losses in the urine. Even when we encourage these patients to drink orange juice and eat bananas (both rich in potassium), we often find the potassium levels low in the blood.

Despite what is known about the risks of diuretics, and even with the knowledge that they will not offer benefit to the 20 percent of all those with hypertension of the squeezing type, many physicians still use this class of medicines first for *all* patients.

Thus, many people like Ron G. are on diuretics unnecessarily. In Ron's example, the diuretic should have been discontinued once it was clear that it was doing no good. On the other hand, for many of these people water pills are a vital part of therapy and should *not* be discontinued. And, as discussed earlier, there are great risks to stopping certain medicines abruptly.

Myth #6:
Salt causes heart attacks.

This is another great salt myth and one worth exploring. The following example is typical:

David M., a forty-six-year-old man recovering from what his doctor said was a "small, warning heart attack," was placed on several medications, including aspirin. His hospital diet was low in cholesterol and low in salt. David's wife told her husband that if he had eaten properly (and avoided salt in the first place) he never would have had the heart attack. When David went home, he found that his wife had filled the kitchen with all of the latest "salt free" products. David was miserable eating food without salt, but decided his health was more important.

David does not have to avoid salt. Eating salty foods did *not* contribute to his heart attack. Only certain people need to avoid salt. This includes people with weak hearts, weak kidneys, and *many* (but *not all*) people with hypertension. David has normal blood pressure. He had a small heart attack, but his heart is otherwise strong. He has blockages in the arteries of his heart, but salt has nothing to do with this problem. Healthy people certainly do *not* have to avoid salt. Although salt is linked to high blood pressure in some people, in reality there are millions of people subjecting themselves to an unpleasant diet for *no reason*. Avoiding salt might even be harmful for some people (such as those with squeezing hypertension).

Like David in the previous example, most people who have had heart attacks will not have any trouble with salt consumption. Yet most cardiac-care units routinely put all patients on salt-restricted diets. *This is irrational!* It is bad enough suffering a heart attack and adjusting to being in a cardiac-care unit, but the adjustment is made worse by being subjected to unpleasant, tasteless food.

Those patients with large heart attacks (and, as a result, with weakened hearts) should be advised to restrict salt intake. But this applies to a minority of patients.

Who Should Avoid Salt?

The same people who should avoid salt will benefit from diuretics. They include:

1. *People with* volume *hypertension*. These people have high blood pressure *because* of the extra salt and water. The pressure can return to normal by restricting dietary salt.

2. *People with congestive heart failure (weak hearts)*. People with weak hearts, such as those who have had large heart attacks, have difficulty pumping even normal amounts of blood. Extra salt and water, by expanding blood volume, will overload the heart. As a result, fluid builds up in the lungs (congestion) and in the tissues of the arms and legs (edema). Avoiding salt is vital to protect the heart and circulation.

3. *People with kidney disease*. The kidneys are responsible for removing extra salt and water. Weak kidneys cannot do the job, and hence salt must be avoided.

4. *Some otherwise healthy people*. Some otherwise healthy people will have a tendency to retain salt, leading to swelling and bloating in different parts of the body. This can be seen in some people after surgery, in people with circulation problems, and frequently in women during menstruation. Although occasionally troublesome and unpleasant, this retention does *not* reflect any serious underlying health problems. Avoiding salt is helpful in preventing the swelling and relieving the symptoms. But it is optional.

The majority of healthy people can eat salt without risk. Patients who have had heart attacks (unless they were large attacks) can eat salt. And people with squeezing hypertension can also eat salt. Too many people avoid it.

Myth #6:
"If I have high blood pressure, I 'must' take medications."

This is an important point to explore. Although doctors typically tell patients that they "must" do many things, they rarely explain what "must" means. Patients have a right to know the risks and benefits and then participate in the decision of whether they are prepared to take medications.

In the example at the beginning of the chapter, Ron was having some unpleasant side effects from his medications. He had mild hypertension and no other medical problems. His doctor told him that he should take prescription medications to prevent a possible heart attack and stroke, implying that it could be a life-and-death issue.

If Ron, who was forty-four years old, was informed that taking medications had a 10 percent *chance* of helping him (by preventing a heart attack or stroke) over the next *twenty years*, he might decide *not* to take them. (There would be a 90 percent chance that he might take medication for twenty years with no result.)

On the other hand, he may decide that a 10 percent chance was worth the expense and side effects of the pills. After all, Ron could never know if he would be one of the 10 percent or not. But at least he would be educated concerning his choice.

Several scientific studies, performed ten to twenty years ago, examined whether treating hypertension made any difference. Patients were randomly assigned to receive medications or to remain untreated. As expected, the patients with the highest levels of blood pressure had the most to gain by therapy. Those patients with more mild hypertension (like Ron) had only a small benefit from drugs.

The actual statistics are revealing:[2]

Diastolic Blood Pressure	Major complications per year	
	NO DRUGS	DRUGS
115–129 (Severe)	30%	2%
105–114 (Moderate)	9.6%	2.5%
95–104 (Mild)	2.5%	2.0%

Patients with severe hypertension had a 30 percent likelihood of having a major complication (either heart attack, stroke, or death) each year. Because treatment with drugs reduced this number to 2 percent a year, the medical community will immediately start therapy in all patients with severe hypertension (with a diastolic blood pressure from 115 to 129). There is a great risk in waiting.

The risk of developing complications with moderate hypertension was found to be 9.6 percent per year, and medical therapy reduced this number to 2.5 percent. Most doctors will also promptly treat this group of patients.

However, with mild hypertension, the difference was found to be less impressive. Those who remained untreated had only a 2.5 percent annual complication rate, which was reduced to 2 percent with drug therapy (a difference of 0.5 percent per year).

Extending this information over a twenty-year period, 50 percent of men with mild hypertension are expected to have a heart attack, stroke, or death if they remain untreated. The use of medications, on the other hand, should reduce this number to 40 percent.

These statistics reflect *all complications:* non-fatal heart attacks and strokes, as well as death. Looking *only* at the influence on survival, it has been estimated that treating mild hypertension, for twenty years, will *save* the lives of 3 men out of every 100. Ninety-seven percent will not have their survival influenced.

When extended to the national level, these numbers become impressive. It has been estimated that there are up to 30 million people with mild hypertension in this country. Saving the lives of 3 percent would represent 900,000 every twenty years, or 45,000 lives a year.

But for any given individual with mild hypertension, the choice is less clear. Taking drugs for twenty years promises only a 3 percent chance of being life-saving and only a 10 percent chance of preventing a complication. There is a large chance the drugs will *not* affect the ultimate outcome, a fact that must be balanced against the expense and side effects of the medications.

It may be important for society to treat everybody with mild hypertension. But if an individual's quality of life is significantly impaired by drugs, then he may have the right to take his chances without therapy. He will, however, accept a 3 percent chance of death during the next twenty years.

While patients with a diastolic blood pressure of 100 to 104 are considered to have mild hypertension, they probably have more to gain by taking medications than those with diastolic pressures of 95 to 99. The presence of other cardiac risk factors—such as smoking, diabetes, and very high cholesterol levels—may also influence the decision to start therapy. In combination with mild hypertension, these factors further add to the risk of complications.

But for those patients who have uncomplicated and mild disease (especially in the 95-to-99 range), immediate drug therapy is not necessary. Weight loss and behavior modification will help some of these patients, and up to 10 percent will get better spontaneously. But even for those who remain with mild hypertension, the risk of waiting, without prescribing drugs, is relatively low.

Myth #8:
"All blood pressure drugs are basically the same. As long as my blood pressure is well controlled, it does not matter what pill I'm taking."

This is an assumption that many doctors and most patients share. There are several dozen drugs available that are effective at lowering blood pressure. This gives a physician a tremendous selection from which to choose.

As long as the drugs used do *not* have unacceptable side effects, we think of them as equally successful if the blood pressure is equally well controlled. Thus, our choice of medication is often based on ease of administration and cost.

Even the Food and Drug Administration has made this assumption. As we mentioned earlier, several scientific studies in the past demonstrated that blood pressure reduction prevented strokes, heart attacks, and death in certain patients. But only a handful of older drugs was used in these studies. Most of the newer drugs have *not* been similarly tested.

The FDA has decided that a drug is acceptable for the treatment of hypertension if it safely and effectively lowers blood pressure. New drugs do *not* have to prove themselves in preventing heart attacks, strokes, and death. All they have to do is lower blood pressure.

By successfully lowering blood pressure, the new drugs are assumed by the FDA to offer the same benefit as the older drugs. Lowering blood pressure is called a surrogate end point.

But can we *assume* that the new drugs are equally effective? Is lowering blood pressure the only thing that matters? A scientific study done in Europe, the results of which were published in the *Journal of the American Medical Association* in 1988, offers some very disturbing results.[3] Indeed, it questions some of our most time-honored assumptions.

The study is called MAPHY (*M*etoprolol *A*therosclerosis *P*revention *H*ypertension). It is the first scientific study to find a significant difference in outcome from the use of two equally effective drugs.

Eleven countries participated in this study, in which over three thousand men with moderately sever hypertension were recruited. This was a *prevention* study; the men chosen had *no* evidence of heart disease at the beginning of the project. The study's objective was to see if the complications associated with high blood pressure could be *prevented*.

Roughly half the men were given a diuretic (hydrochlorothiazide, HCTZ) as their first drug. The other half of the men were given a beta-blocker (metoprolol) as their first drug. Both types of drugs are commonly given to patients with high blood pressure.

Diuretics lower blood pressure by reducing the volume of water in the circulation. Consequently they are called water pills. Beta-blockers have two desirable actions—they block the action of adrenaline in the body, and they block the release of renin from the kidneys. Both of these effects contribute to lower blood pressure.

In MAPHY, if the first drug administered was *not* successful in controlling blood pressure, others were added as needed. Men in the beta-blocker group were not allowed to receive a diuretic as their second drug, and vice versa. Otherwise, many men in the two groups would end up taking the same combination of drugs: both a diuretic and a beta-blocker.

At the end of the study, 50 percent of the men in each group were controlled by either the diuretic or beta-blocker alone, while the other 50 percent of men required at least a second drug.

Blood pressure was equally well controlled in the two groups, as seen here:

MAPHY

	HCTZ	METOPROLOL
number of men	1,625	1,609
initial BP (before drugs)	167/108	167/108
final BP (after drugs)	143/89	143/89

Hypertension therapy with either HCTZ or metoprolol resulted in equally acceptable control of blood pressure. At the end of the study there was no difference between the two groups besides the choice of the first drug. Therefore, according to our assumption, the men in each group should do equally well.

But they did not!

After treating the men for four years, the number of deaths in the metoprolol group was nearly 50 percent lower than in the HCTZ group.

MAPHY: 4 YEAR SURVIVAL

	HCTZ	METOPROLOL
number of men	1,625	1,609
number of deaths	54	28

The metoprolol group *should* have had the same number of deaths as the HCTZ group, since blood pressure was equally controlled. But there were fewer deaths in this group. During four years of treatment, 26 men (out of 1,609) had their lives *saved* simply because their blood pressure was treated primarily with metoprolol instead of HCTZ.

It is not known why treatment with metoprolol had better results than with HCTZ. Metoprolol has been demonstrated to prevent death in other groups of people, such as those who have been sent home from the hospital after having had a heart attack. The drug is believed to offer a chemical protection to the heart. Therefore, it is possible that, besides lowering blood pressure, metoprolol offers patients benefits beyond HCTZ.

Twenty-six men out of 1,609 (the number who had their lives saved by metoprolol therapy during a four-year period) represents 1.6 percent of the total group. If we extend this to the 30 million people with mild to moderate hypertension in the United States, the total number of lives saved can approach over 100,000 per year.

However, we cannot fully extend the study's results to all people with high blood pressure. The MAPHY study involved: 1. men only; 2. men between the ages of forty and sixty-four; 3. men with moderate hypertension; and 4. men without preexisting heart disease. This is a very specific group of people and, strictly speaking, the results apply only to this group.

But an important point has been made by the study: equal control of blood pressure does not necessarily mean equal survival.

Yet even after the availability of these results, diuretics (like HCTZ) are still the most common first drug used to treat hypertension in the United States. MAPHY suggests that many of these patients would do better on metoprolol.

Unfortunately, metoprolol can't be safely given to all patients. It can worsen congestive heart failure, and can cause asthma attacks. There are many other drugs currently available for the treatment of hypertension. We do not know how they would compare to metoprolol, if studied. But a major challenge has been presented. We can no longer assume that all medications will offer the same benefit.

Myth #9:
"My blood pressure is too low!"

Some people who are in excellent health become concerned when their doctor tells them that they have low blood pressure. But this is usually not a medical problem. In fact it is actually healthy to have lower-than-average blood pressure.

> Linda P., a fifty-year-old woman whose blood pressure was found to be 90/60, has never been significantly dizzy and has never fainted. But because of her low blood pressure she has been afraid to be active.

Linda has a naturally low blood pressure. Because she has no symptoms, her blood pressure is *not* too low *for her*. In fact, Linda has a lower-than-average risk for a stroke and a heart attack because of this chronically depressed blood pressure.

Although a good thing for most people, a blood pressure of 90/60 *might* be poorly tolerated in others. This is especially likely in those with chronic hypertension.

Julie K., a seventy-nine-year-old woman, went to the emergency room because she had chest pains and difficulty breathing. Her blood pressure was found to be 210/120.

She was given several pills, and within one hour it was down. Julie started to feel "much better," but the medicine caused her blood pressure to continue to fall.

Thirty minutes later Julie became very confused. She started to undress, and did not know where she was. She began to speak incoherently. Her blood pressure was found to be 110/80.

Julie was put flat in bed, and intravenous fluids were administered (these efforts increase blood pressure). Soon Julie's blood pressure increased to 150/95, and she started to "clear up," slowly regaining her orientation.

In Julie's case, the rapid fall in her blood pressure was too much for her. Although a blood pressure of 110/80 is perfectly normal for most people, it was insufficient for Julie.

Julie's circulation was accustomed to working at a very high blood pressure, which helps to push blood up to her brain. An abrupt fall in this pressure proved to be poorly tolerated. Julie became confused when her blood pressure fell to 110/80, whereas most other people have no trouble handling a blood pressure this low.

Other symptoms of low blood pressure include dizziness (the most common symptom), weakness, and fainting. These symptoms have many causes, and their presence does not automatically imply that blood pressure is too low. But if the blood pressure is depressed, and a patient has these symptoms, they are probably related.

There is no absolute number that represents a low blood pressure for everybody. It is a very individual situation. In the absence of symptoms, a low blood pressure is usually a good thing.

∧∧∧∧∧

CHAPTER THREE

Bypass Surgery

Heart bypass surgery has captured the imagination of the public. It is currently the most common major operation performed in the United States (more than 250,000 bypass surgeries are performed each year). The surgery is sometimes life-saving. Often it is not. And it is always frightening.

For many, it is the most significant medical event in their lives. Many view it as a rebirth, and are psychologically strengthened by their perception of having brand new heart arteries. Others never fully recover from the emotional trauma of the event. And there are, of course, physical complications of the procedure.

The psychological implications of bypass surgery contribute to the genesis of many myths and misconceptions. People have remarkable fantasies concerning the mechanics of the operation itself, and most of these are inaccurate. And almost every patient feels that the surgery has saved *his* life.

Often this is not the case. There have been critics who claim that many bypass operations are unnecessary. But this is not the only consideration.

The medical and emotional issues aside, there are also tremendous financial implications to bypass surgery. It is a multibillion-dollar-a-year business. And it is a procedure now being challenged by a newer concept: balloon angioplasty.

Bypass surgery and balloon angioplasty are both procedures designed to improve the flow of blood through the coronary arteries. There are three such arteries that run on the surface of the heart, serving as fuel lines, normally delivering up to four times *more* blood than the heart muscle needs.

When deposits of cholesterol grow on the inside of these arteries, the amount of blood that passes through is reduced and the heart gets less fuel. Minor blockages (with less than a 50 percent reduction of the diameter of the artery) will still allow a surplus of blood to reach the heart muscle.

But as arteries get more narrowed, the heart begins to suffer. The lack of blood (and oxygen) results in chest pains (most commonly during physical activity), which we call angina. Furthermore, these cholesterol blockages can, abruptly, become covered by the formation of a blood clot, resulting in the complete occlusion of the artery. This causes a heart attack.

A bypass operation is designed to fix these blockages and restore normal blood flow to the heart muscle. There are three goals to bypass surgery: 1. to relieve chest pain; 2. to prevent heart attacks; and 3. to prevent death.

Before a bypass operation can be performed, a surgeon requires a precise map of the arteries and their blockages. The test that supplies this information is called a cardiac catheterization or angiogram. Cardiac catheterization is greatly misunderstood.

Myth #1:
A cardiac catheterization is an extremely painful and dangerous test.

This is a common perception. Patients frequently become anxious when told they need a cardiac catheterization, anticipating pain and a dangerous procedure. Most discover their fears to be worse than the actual test.

In cardiac catheterization, a small needle is placed through the skin into the femoral artery, which is situated in the groin and which supplies blood to the leg. Alternatively, an artery supplying the arm can be used. Local anesthesia is used to numb the skin. Once the needle is within the artery, a long, but narrow, hollow plastic tube (called a catheter) is threaded into the circulatory system. This entire phase of the procedure usually causes a moment of "pinching" pain.

Under X-ray guidance, the catheter is moved up through the circulatory system (through the aorta) until it reaches the arteries supplying the heart muscle (the coronary arteries). This is entirely painless; there is no sensation on the inside of blood vessels.

When the catheter reaches the coronary arteries, contrast material (commonly called dye) is rapidly injected through the catheter. A movie is taken with an X-ray camera, recording the flow of the contrast material down the inside of the arteries. Blockages are readily identified and measured. All three arteries are studied. The need and nature of bypass surgery are defined.

Some risk does accompany a cardiac catheterization. There is a one-in-one-thousand chance of experiencing a heart at-

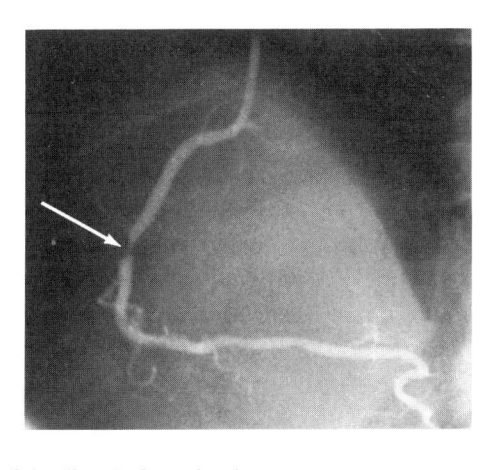

Photograph of Cardiac Catheterization
Injecting contrast material down the artery reveals a 95% blockage.

tack, stroke, or death *because* of the procedure. As the site of entry, the femoral artery can be damaged by the catheter. In extremely rare cases, patients have lost a leg because of this injury.

The contrast material is toxic to the kidneys. This is especially true for people with diabetes, and a very small number of patients require dialysis after the test. Finally, some patients will experience an allergic reaction to the contrast material. Patients with a previous allergy to iodine are particularly vulnerable.

Although these complications are grim, they are also extremely rare. And, most important, there is also a risk involved in *not* performing the test. We usually recommend a cardiac catheterization to patients who have potentially severe heart disease, and who are at an increased risk for experiencing a heart attack, stroke, or even death *without* intervention. Cardiac catheterization is a necessary step before bypass surgery can be performed. The test is justified when the benefits outweigh the risks.

Some patients undergo a cardiac catheterization because it is uncertain whether they have heart disease:

> Martha D., a fifty-two-year-old woman, was admitted to the hospital with severe chest pains. Her electrocardiogram (EKG) remained normal, and she showed no signs of having had a heart attack. She continued to have episodes of chest pains despite advancing doses of heart medications.
>
> Martha underwent a cardiac catheterization, and was found to have *normal* coronary arteries. There were no blockages, and the pains were not emanating from her heart.
>
> Although the cause of her chest pains was not determined, it was clear that Martha had a normal heart. Her cardiac medications were stopped, and she was discharged. An evaluation of her pain was continued as an outpatient.

For patients like Martha, a cardiac catheterization can prove there is *no* heart disease, an important use of this test.

After the cardiac catheterization the surgeon can proceed, if clinically indicated, with bypass surgery. This brings us to the myths of the surgery itself.

Myth #2:
During bypass surgery the blockage in the artery of the heart is removed.

This is the most common myth about the mechanics of bypass surgery. Most people do *not* have a clear understanding of what is involved in the procedure. The basic concept is found in the name of the operation: "bypass."

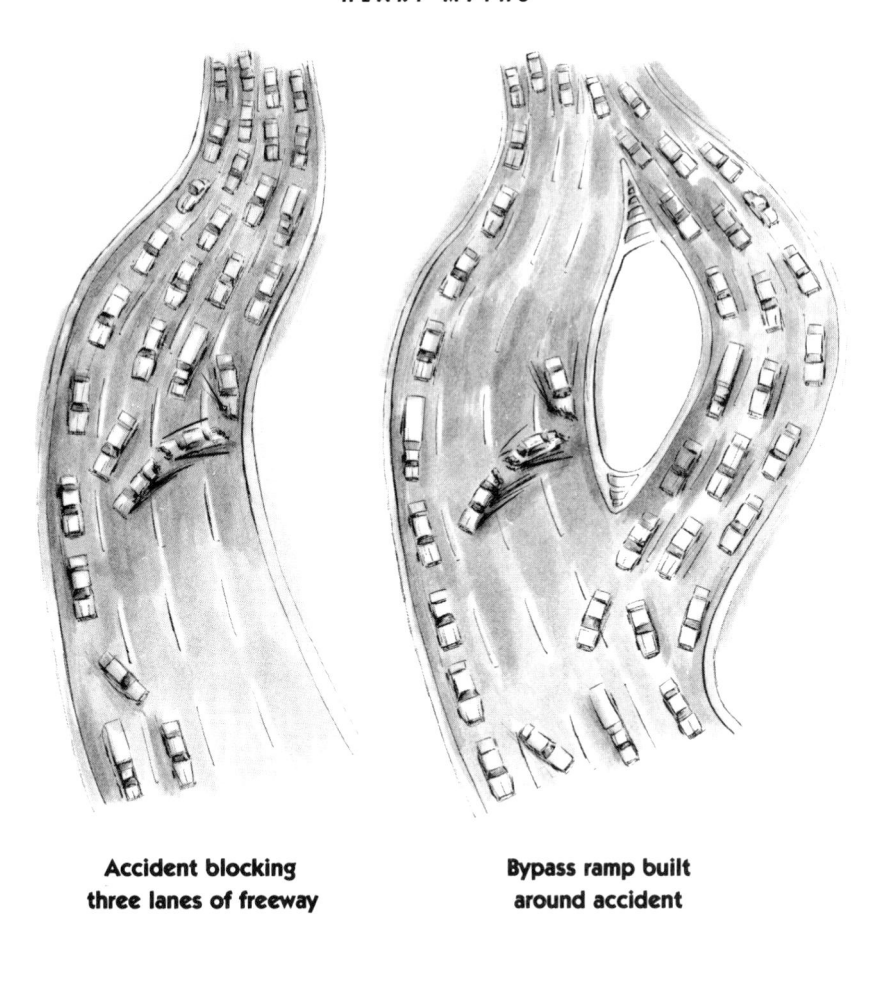

**Accident blocking
three lanes of freeway**

**Bypass ramp built
around accident**

Consider, as an analogy, a normal freeway with four lanes of traffic moving smoothly in one direction. If an accident were to occur and block three lanes of the freeway, leaving only one lane open, this would cause traffic congestion.

The cars back up for miles, slowly moving past the accident just as blood backs up in a blocked artery. In automobile accidents, we remove the cars that are blocking traffic. But it is not so easy to remove a blockage out of an artery in the heart. (As discussed later, the relatively new approach of balloon angioplasty does, in effect, remove the blockage from the artery.)

There is another way to get traffic moving, however. We can build a new ramp to divert traffic, allowing most cars to go around or bypass the blockage.

Some cars will continue to move in the original direction and squeeze past the accident. But the new ramp has become the major route of traffic.

Though impractical from the perspective of our highway maintenance departments, this solution is analogous to what is done to the heart during a bypass operation. Deposits of cholesterol block blood flow in the coronary arteries, causing a backup. A bypass operation is designed to place a new tube (or graft) into the circulation of the heart to bypass the blockage. One end of the graft is attached to the aorta (which is the major freeway of the body), the other to the coronary artery beyond the site of the blockage. The bypass creates an alternate route of blood flow to the heart muscle.

There are two types of tubes (grafts) commonly used for bypass surgery:

1. VEIN FROM THE LEG:
The most common tubes used for a bypass operation are segments of vein (the saphenous vein) cut out of the leg. With a saphenous vein graft (abbreviated SVG), the ends of this venous segment are attached to the aorta and the coronary artery, respectively. Through the SVG, blood flow can bypass the narrowed segment and supply the heart muscle with its demand for fuel.

There are some consequences to removing a segment of the saphenous vein, the major route through which blood leaves the leg. After the segment of vein is removed, the remaining ends are literally tied off, interrupting the flow of blood in that vein. Blood enters the leg through the arteries easily, but does not exit easily. Blood builds up with increasing pressure, and this results in fluid being squeezed out of the circulation into the tissues. This fluid (called edema) causes the legs to swell, and is a common problem after bypass surgery.

Eventually tiny new veins, called collaterals, grow in the leg and allow blood to leave with greater ease. Often these collaterals normalize the flow of blood from the leg and relieve the edema.

Not all saphenous veins are suitable for use during bypass surgery. In the case of people with severe varicose veins, (a condition which grossly distorts the flow of blood), the saphenous veins cannot be used.

2. ARTERY FROM THE CHEST:

The other common tubes used for bypass surgery are the two special arteries that are already in the chest: the internal mammary arteries (IMA). These arteries supply blood to the inside wall of the chest, on both the right and left sides, and are otherwise *not* very important in most people.

Unlike a vein from the leg, the internal mammary artery is *not* removed, but, instead, is left in the chest. The IMA is cut in half, and one end is attached to the blocked coronary artery. It is inserted "downstream" of the blockage, and thus redirects blood that had previously flowed to the chest wall, to the heart muscle instead. The remaining end of the IMA is tied off.

Internal mammary artery grafts are more durable than venous grafts, and last much longer. Approximately 90 percent to 95 percent of them are functional ten years after surgery, whereas only 50 percent of venous grafts last that long.

Unfortunately, there are just two IMAs in the chest, and

most heart surgeons will use only one of them. The interruption of one of these arteries does not have a big impact in a patient; but cutting both can lead to a noticeable reduction of blood flow to the chest wall, in turn resulting in numbness of the overlying skin and an increased likelihood of developing a wound infection after surgery. Consequently, most surgeons are reluctant to use both IMAs, and a combination of SVGs and IMAs used in most surgical procedures. Furthermore, IMAs, which are themselves arteries, are not always in suitable condition for use as grafts in bypass surgery. They can have their own atherosclerotic narrowings, and hence might be too diseased for use in the heart. This is a common problem in the elderly. Veins typically remain free of atherosclerosis, and hence more available.

The IMA is smaller than the saphenous vein, and working with it requires greater technical skill and more time in the operating room. Because time is often a crucial factor, the IMA is not commonly used during emergency operations.

In very rare cases, neither the saphenous vein nor the internal mammary artery can be used:

Ruth S. is an eighty-one-year-old woman suffering from uncontrollable chest pains despite maximal medications. She underwent cardiac catheterization that revealed severe blockages in all three of the major arteries of her heart. Initially refusing to consider an operation, Ruth returned to the hospital two days later with severe chest pains and requested surgery.

Ironically, after examining her, the surgeon exclaimed, "I cannot operate!" Ruth had profound varicose veins in both her legs, making the saphenous veins virtually unusable as grafts. Likewise, the IMAs in an eighty-one-year-old are usually too diseased (with their own atherosclerosis) for use in bypass surgery. The surgeon could not justify operating on so elderly a patient with such poor odds of success.

There are two other tubes available but rarely used as bypass grafts. Veins can be removed from the arms, but they tend to do very poorly, lasting a very short time. Additionally, intravenous (IV) lines and the drawing of blood for tests commonly damage these veins, making them even more difficult to use. In the rare circumstance that a vein must be taken from an arm, it is best to have anticipated and minimized the puncturing of these veins.

There are artificial tubes available for bypass surgery, but they are very rarely used. As foreign bodies, they tend both to clot and become infected more easily than natural veins or arteries.

All grafts, regardless of their type, provide an alternative route for blood to flow through the arteries of the heart. The original artery in the heart is otherwise untouched and the blockage is left in place. It is literally bypassed.

Blood can still squeeze past the blockage, but is overshadowed by the amount of flow down the bypass graft. In some patients the blockage will close off entirely, leaving the heart entirely dependent on the graft for blood flow. In these cases, the durability of the graft assumes an even greater importance.

Myth #3:
The more blood vessels that are bypassed, the more
impressive the operation is.

"Mine was a *quadruple!*" Often this is stated with a curious pride, as though a "quadruple" is somehow more *impressive* than a single, double, or triple bypass; that the ordeal of a quadruple bypass is that much greater.

However, the operative risk is *not* appreciably different for a single, double, triple, or quadruple bypass. The only dif-

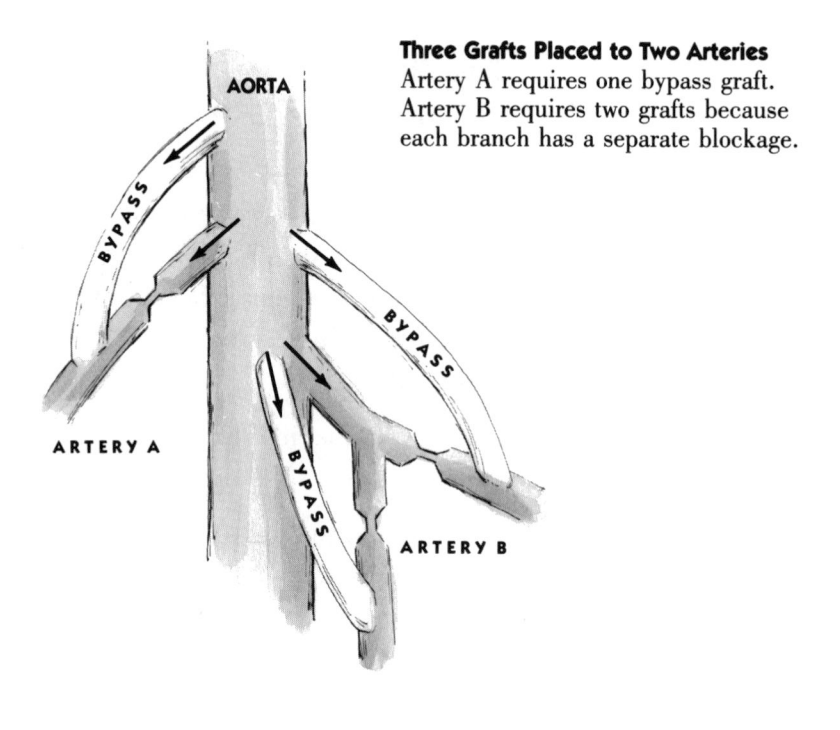

Three Grafts Placed to Two Arteries
Artery A requires one bypass graft.
Artery B requires two grafts because
each branch has a separate blockage.

ference is in the number of narrowed arteries that are repaired.

There are only three coronary arteries that supply blood to the heart. But some people require up to four or five grafts during their surgery. This apparent paradox is easily explained.

Each of the three arteries to the heart has several branches of different sizes, which can each have their own blockages. Thus, any given artery can require more than one bypass graft: one to the main artery and one to the major branch. This is demonstrated in the diagram above:

It is not easier to have one's chest cut open for a single bypass than for a quadruple bypass. The mechanics of surgery are the same, involving the following steps:

Basic Steps of
Coronary Artery Bypass Surgery

1. Anesthesia is administered (called induction) and a tube is placed down the throat to pump air into the lungs. This is often the *most dangerous* step of surgery, because there can be dramatic changes of blood pressure and heart rate when anesthetic agents are first given.

2. An incision is made down the middle of the chest straight through to the breastbone.

3. An electric saw is used to cut through the breastbone, opening up the chest cavity. Retractors are used to spread the ribs apart (this is one reason there is so much chest pain *after* surgery; the chest has been greatly traumatized by the spreading of the ribs).

4. An incision is made down one or both legs, to obtain the necessary number of saphenous venous segments.

5. Special tubes are inserted into the chambers of the heart and into the aorta. These are attached to an external device (called the pump). The pump will work for the heart during surgery, as the heart will be stopped (because it is not practical to work on a moving target).

6. The heart is cooled to 53° F. with ice water and then is literally stopped by an infusion of a potassium solution (which causes temporary paralysis of the heart muscle). The cool temperature protects the muscle while it is not working. The external pump is activated, then moves blood through the body. The heart is not beating.

7. The arteries that require a bypass graft are located on

the outside surface of the heart. The heart is not cut open (another common myth). The ends of the venous segments are respectively attached to the aorta and the diseased coronary arteries. And, if used, the internal mammary artery is divided, and one end is attached to a coronary artery.

8. When the work is completed the heart is warmed back to body temperature (98.6° F.), the potassium solution is rinsed away, and the heart is restarted with an electric shock. After it starts beating, the tubes to the external pump are removed, and the heart takes over the work of the circulation.

9. The chest wall is closed with loops of wire, and the skin of the chest is sutured together.

The operation is always a major ordeal, on average lasting from four to six hours. If only one artery requires repair, the operation is a single bypass. If four arteries are repaired, then the operation is called a quadruple bypass. But there is otherwise no difference in what is required for a single or quadruple bypass operation. The risk and trauma of the operation are the same. More grafts mean that there was more extensive underlying disease. But this is not necessarily something in which to take pride.

Myth #4:
After a bypass the heart is "as good as new."

Unfortunately, this is *not* true. The heart is improved, but is not as good as new. The grafts (new tubes) return normal blood flow to the previously deprived heart muscle. The heart once again receives enough oxygen and nutrients from the blood to maintain its energy requirements. Chest pain (angina) is thus eliminated in most patients.

But the damaged heart muscle cannot be repaired and some arteries are too sick for bypass grafting. Furthermore, the benefits of surgery do not last forever; in fact, the majority of grafts will be functional for less than twelve years. The bypass operation is not a "cure."

Limitations of Bypass Surgery

1. *Damaged heart muscle will remain damaged after bypass surgery.* Dead and scarred muscle (from a previous heart attack) will *not* get better. Some regions of the heart that had been stunned by the stress of limited blood flow will beat more strongly after surgery. But other areas can never improve.

Life expectancy depends significantly on the strength of the heart muscle. A weak heart is bad. A very weak heart is even worse. And a bypass operation, in general, has little if any effect on heart muscle strength.

Some people will experience a heart attack during the surgery itself, resulting in even greater damage to the heart muscle. This is an uncommon, but serious, risk of surgery.

Sam M., a sixty-one-year-old man, had had a large heart attack ten years ago, which was immediately followed by a bypass operation. In recent months he developed recurrent chest pain, which, in spite of medications, was limiting his ability to perform day-to-day activities. His doctor strongly recommended a second bypass operation.

The second operation was prolonged and complicated because the inside of his chest was heavily scarred from the original bypass. As a result of this stress, Sam had another, moderately large, heart attack *during* surgery.

Although his arteries were repaired, and his chest pain was eliminated, Sam now had severe shortness of breath, which was more limiting than his preoperative symptoms. His heart had been severely damaged by the cumulative effects of two heart attacks. He died six months after the operation from heart failure.

2. *Some of the narrowed arteries can* not *be fixed by bypass surgery.*

Jack P., a sixty-year-old man, had four significant blockages in the arteries of his heart. He was told by his cardiologist that he needed a quadruple bypass. After the operation, however, his surgeon told him that only two of the arteries had been repaired. One of the remaining arteries was too small, and the other was too diffusely diseased to permit placement of a bypass graft. The surgeon still considered the operation to be "a success." The circulation was clearly improved by the operation, but it was obviously not as good as new.

Bypass grafts must be attached to the recipient artery downstream of the blockage. In some cases this is not technically possible because the artery is too small, or because it has diffuse blockages throughout its entire length.

3. *Blockages continue to develop and grow in the arteries of the heart during the years after a bypass operation.* New blockages can appear in arteries that were normal at the time of the bypass operation, in arteries that have already been bypassed (but even further downstream of the insertion of the graft), and in the bypass grafts themselves.

Atherosclerosis takes decades to develop in the arteries of

the heart. Thirty to forty years of smoking, a high cholesterol level, high blood pressure, diabetes, and wear and tear all contribute to the slow but progressive process of "hardening of the arteries." However, the disease accelerates after a bypass operation, with new blockages developing as early as three to four years after the surgery. In fact, more than 50 percent of arteries that have been bypassed will reveal new evidence of disease one year after the operation.

4. *The bypass grafts can totally shut down, with a complete blockage.* This is the most troubling postoperative problem. Ten years after the operation a high percentage of venous grafts are in trouble.

Approximately 30 percent to 50 percent will be totally occluded, and an additional 30 percent will have developed significant narrowings limiting the flow of blood to the heart. Thus, the majority of bypass grafts will not be functional a decade after surgery. The IMAs have a more successful chance (90 percent to 95 percent) of remaining functional during this time period. Even so, many patients will require a second operation.

Chuck S., a fifty-year-old man who had a double bypass nine years ago, developed recurrent chest pain. A cardiac catheterization was performed, revealing that the two grafts, each helping a blocked coronary artery were now completely occluded. The third artery (which had not been bypassed in the original operation) had developed a new, and significant, blockage.

Chuck was told that he needed another bypass operation. He was stunned. "I thought that the bypass fixed everything. No one told me that I would need another one!"

Unfortunately, Chuck faces a much higher risk for sudden death without another operation. Nearly 2 million people in the United States have already had bypass operations. During the next decade many of these people will find themselves in the same situation, facing a second bypass operation (called a "re-op" in medical parlance.).

A second bypass operation is usually more difficult than the first, because scar tissue forms in the chest after the initial operation, and because often the best veins have already been taken from the legs. As a result, the operative risks are somewhat higher. Surgeons try to avoid performing second procedures, but some patients have serious recurrent disease and clearly require another repair.

Myth #5:
Bypass surgery prevents heart attacks.

Most people are surprised to learn that this is not always true.

Harry L., a seventy-three-year-old man with exertional chest pain, had a stress test that strongly suggested that he had heart disease. A cardiac catheterization revealed blockages in two out of three of the major arteries of his heart. The blockage in one artery had resulted in a 95 percent narrowing, while the other was narrowed by 80 percent. Harry had never had a heart attack, and the strength of his heart was normal.

His doctor advised a bypass operation: "You don't want to have a heart attack, do you? That ninety-five-percent narrowing is just waiting to close off. You should have your operation as soon as possible."

Harry may have a heart attack one day, but bypass surgery will not lower this risk.

Just because an artery is 95 percent narrowed does not mean that it is "just waiting" to close off. Many of the arteries will remain stable for years. It is inappropriate to make these patients feel that they are walking time bombs.

Furthermore, the stress of surgery can *cause* a heart attack to occur in the operating room. And heart attacks can occur in bypass patients months to years later, despite the operation. Indeed, the net balance reveals that bypass surgery does not *statistically* prevent heart attacks. It is *not* certain that Harry would be better off with an operation.

This applies also to patients with "unstable angina," a syndrome of worsening chest pain. Harry had "exertional" chest pain; that occurs only during activity, in a stable and predictable pattern. However, some patients experience progressive worsening of their symptoms, characterized by more frequent episodes of pain brought on by less and less activity. This pattern continues to crescendo, with prolonged episodes of chest pain finally occurring at rest. The pattern of "unstable angina" strongly suggests that a heart attack will occur in the near future.

Bypass surgery does not necessarily prevent heart attacks even in these patients. The available data suggest that surgery is as likely to *cause* a heart attack as it is to *prevent* one. Yet patients with unstable angina are frequently advised to have bypass surgery "to prevent a heart attack."

Patients with unstable angina often require enormous amounts of medication, and in some cases, even the most aggressive medical therapy fails to control chest pain. Bypass surgery becomes the only way to achieve a relief of symptoms and a reduction of medications. But we cannot claim that we are preventing heart attacks.

Myth #6:
Your bypass operation has saved your life!

Almost all patients feel that bypass surgery has saved *their lives*. But this is not the case for the majority of people. The bypass operation represents a tremendous mental and physical ordeal, and is also quite expensive (costing roughly $40,000). It is easy to understand a patient's need to justify undergoing the procedure.

Additionally, the surgery can be fatal. There is a 1 percent to 2 percent chance of dying during a routine bypass operation. The risks increase from 3 percent to 25 percent with advancing age (generally over eighty years old), general poor health, weak heart, and recent heart attacks. Those who require more complex cardiac surgery, such as a valve replacement in addition to the bypass, are at even higher risk.

As a result, patients are generally grateful to have survived the operation. Because they faced death, there is a sense of having had their lives saved. But this does *not* mean that the surgery was life-saving. The patient faced the risk of death by having the operation in the first place. The more important question is whether surgery prolongs life beyond simply taking medications. Is Harry L., in the previous example, likely to live longer because he had a bypass operation? Or should he have remained on medications?

Several large scientific studies examining these issues have been performed in both Europe and the United States. Relatively young, healthy, and stable patients with heart disease were randomly assigned to have either a bypass operation or to remain on medications. The patients were carefully monitored over many years. Did surgery keep people alive longer?

A well-publicized study called CASS[1] (Coronary Artery Surgery Study), conducted in the United States, randomized 780 middle-aged patients to either bypass surgery or to medical therapy. After six years of follow-up, the survival rate in both groups was very similar: surgical group—92 percent; medical group—90 percent.

Surgery did not significantly influence survival. Approximately 10 percent of patients died within both the medical and surgical groups during the six years of follow-up. *Of note, operative mortality was included in the surgical statistics.*

Total mortality was rather low in both groups (only 1 percent to 2 percent died a year) because the patients selected for this study were relatively young and otherwise healthy heart patients. Scientists are *not* sure if these results can be applied to older, sicker, and more symptomatic patients.

However, the study delivered a clear message. Surgery does not have a significant overall influence on survival. Each year 1 percent to 2 percent of patients died, whether or not surgery was performed.

Although surgery did not prolong survival for the entire group, some *subgroups* of patients were more likely to receive a benefit, such as those with the most number of blockages in their hearts.

We can count how many of the three arteries in the heart have significant blockages. Simply stated, patients have either one- two- or three-vessel diseases. Those with three blockages have more heart attacks and death than those with fewer blockages. Bypass surgery has potentially more to offer these higher risk patients.

The following survival data is available from the CASS study:

# OF ARTERIES WITH BLOCKAGES	CASS 6-YEAR SURVIVAL	
	MEDICAL	SURGICAL
1	93%	96%
2	94%	95%
3	89%	93%

The survival of patients who have either one or two arteries blocked is very good with medications alone (93 percent and 94 percent, respectively, during the six years of follow-up). Surgery does *not* appreciably improve the chance of survival for these subgroups.

Harry, in the previous example, had two vessels narrowed. His chance of surviving six years was excellent regardless of his decision to have an operation. Statistically, his medical survival would have been as good as his surgical survival. Surgery cannot be called life-saving in this case.

There is a moderately improved surgical survival rate in those patients with three-vessel disease. The six-year medical survival is only 89 percent, whereas the surgical survival is 93 percent. This is not a big difference. But not all patients with three-vessel disease are equal. Some are clearly sicker than others.

Some patients with three-vessel disease will do very well on an exercise test, whereas others have extreme changes in the electrocardiogram after performing very little exercise (a very bad result). This is an important distinction. A very abnormal result implies that the blockages have a bigger impact than in those with a good exercise result.

Patients with three-vessel disease and very abnormal exercise testing form a subgroup for whom surgery imparts a big improvement in six-year survival as compared to medical therapy.

CASS
6-YEAR SURVIVAL

	MEDICAL	SURGICAL
3 arteries with blockages and very abnormal exercise test result	58%	81%

This subgroup of patients clearly received benefit from bypass surgery. The medical mortality is quite significant for these patients. Medical therapy kept only 58 percent alive for six years, whereas surgery kept 81 percent alive. In other words, 23 percent of men survived the six years of the study *because* they were randomly assigned to have surgery instead of simply taking medication.

It is interesting to note that, in this group of patients, surgery prevented sudden cardiac death, but it did *not* prevent heart attacks. This may sound like a strange distinction, but some people die suddenly (from an abrupt change in the electrical activity of the heart) without suffering from a heart attack (which is the death of heart muscle). Bypass surgery can save lives without preventing heart attacks.

A fifty-year-old man in this subgroup would almost certainly choose surgery (when faced with a 23 percent chance of having his life saved). But an eighty-year-old might find that the ordeal of surgery is not justified by the benefits, and accordingly might decide to take his chances with medications. A 23 percent risk over six years may not seem too important to someone that age, and a physician cannot make this judgment for the patient. The patient should be told the actual risks and benefits of surgery and then make the decision with the help of the doctor.

Another subgroup of patients that benefits from surgery is that with three-vessel disease and a weak heart. Previous damage from a heart attack leaves the heart weaker than normal. These patients have already sustained damage and cannot afford to suffer more loss of heart muscle. Having blockages in all three coronary arteries puts them at added risk.

CASS
6-YEAR SURVIVAL

	MEDICAL	SURGICAL
3 arteries with blockages and weak hearts	65%	88%

This group of patients is also more likely to be alive in six years because of bypass surgery. Whereas 65 percent of those treated only with medicines survived, 88 percent of those who had bypass surgery survived. Surgery is clearly desirable for these patients, although the majority of those on whom we operate will *not* have their lives saved. Since we can't predict in advance who will be one of the 23 percent who are saved, we operate on the entire group.

There are dangers in misrepresenting the risks and benefits of medical and surgical therapy. Occasionally some patients reach distorted conclusions. Consider the following example:

John G., a fifty-eight-year-old man, told his doctor that he had chest "tightness" during periods of exertion. An exercise test strongly suggested that John had severe heart disease. An ensuing cardiac catheterization revealed very severe blockage in all three of his coronary arteries. John was told that he should have the problem "fixed" by surgery.

John flatly refused to have the operation. His doctor warned him that he would probably die, and that this was a life-or-death issue. But John refused to face the facts and left his doctor, refusing to return.

Six years later John called his doctor to say, "I told you so! I'm still alive!"

John had taken a gamble with his life that paid off. But he survived because of the odds. If, during those six years, John had participated in an exercise or dietary program, taken fish-oil pills, or even meditated, he might choose to believe such therapy was the reason he survived. He could further be exploited: "A dramatic example of a person whose life was saved . . . by Product X. His doctors said he would be dead without an operation, but we kept him alive!"

John had had blockages in all three arteries, and he had a very abnormal exercise test result. As a result, the odds tell us that he stood a 58 percent chance of surviving the seven years without surgery, and an 81 percent chance of survival with it. He misunderstood his doctor, and his doctor to some extent misrepresented the benefits of surgery. Bypass surgery does not guarantee survival, and declining surgery does not mean certain death. It comes down to basic statistics. *There are no guarantees, only choices.*

Myth #7:
"I'm too old to have bypass surgery."

Often patients believe they are too old for the rigors of bypass surgery.

Helen J., an eighty-three-year-old woman in a cardiac care unit, had worsening chest pain. Her cardiac catheterization revealed several blockages in all three arteries of her heart. Her heart had been moderately weakened from a heart attack earlier that week. She was on very large doses of cardiac medications, given both orally and intravenously, and on sedatives. But she was still having up to three or four episodes of angina a day. Surgery was recommended by her doctors, but Helen said, "I'm too old and too sick for surgery. Let me rest several days and regain my strength."

This is common concern of the elderly, but, surprisingly, age is not a very important factor. Older patients can do extremely well with bypass surgery. The operative mortality can be as low as 5 percent to 6 percent for uncomplicated patients in their early eighties, but as high as 25 percent for more complex cases.

For patients like Helen, bypass surgery is a very survivable procedure. Furthermore, sooner is better than later. Patients often want to wait until they feel better before having their surgery. But for unstable patients this is not always possible. They may get worse by waiting.

There is no evidence that Helen would live longer if she had surgery. At age eighty-three, surgery can not be assumed life-saving. And surgery is *not* expected to prevent another heart attack. But surgery may be necessary to relieve symptoms.

Helen was having uncontrollable symptoms. She could not possibly go home taking either the intravenous drugs or the massive doses of her oral medications. And even with these drugs the pain was unmanageable. She had no other realistic alternative. Bypass surgery was the only hope for pain control.

The surgical complications are indeed greater for octogenarians. The postoperative hospital stay is significantly longer. The incidence of infection (in the lungs and surgical wounds) is greater. Recovery can take months.

However, despite the increased risks of surgery, some clinical circumstances, like those of Helen, force the surgical hand in these more elderly patients. The risks of surgery are hence outweighed by the benefits (quality of life, control of pain).

Myth #8:
Most bypass surgery is unnecessary.

Scientific studies have indicated that most people will not live longer, and heart attacks will not necessarily be prevented, because of bypass surgery. Hence, the operation is often called "unnecessary." But this judgment may be incorrect.

Not all benefits are measured by survival statistics. Many patients will live *better* because of their operation. Symptoms of angina are enormously relieved by bypass surgery. The need for taking medications is often dramatically reduced and the ability to live an active and productive life is enhanced.

Greg S., a forty-two-year-old construction worker with angina, took three different heart medications, yet still experienced chest pain once or twice a day. His exercise test was interpreted as "not too bad." But because his life-style was impaired, he underwent an angiogram to see if anything could be fixed.

He was found to have blockages in two of the three coronary arteries. The blockages were not ideal for repair by the relatively new procedure of balloon angioplasty.

Greg elected to have surgery, which was successful in eliminating his chest pain and his need for taking medications (except for one aspirin a day). He returned to work two months after his operation, feeling much better than before the bypass operation.

Was this operation unnecessary? Greg is not expected to live longer because of the surgery. But his *quality of life* has been greatly improved.

Unfortunately, these benefits are not likely to last forever. Greg faces a 20 percent chance of developing recurrent angina during the first year after his surgery, and a 50 percent likelihood of experiencing recurrent symptoms a decade later. Closure of the grafts and the development of new blockages threaten long-term surgical results. Greg may even require a second operation sometime in the future (which has on average a 10 percent operative mortality).

We cannot think of bypass surgery as a permanent cure, or as only a "once in a lifetime" deal for everyone, especially when operating on people in their forties and fifties. It may be more realistic to think of surgery as a temporary repair of coronary artery disease, lasting an average ten years.

There is also an immediate 1 percent to 2 percent gamble (operative mortality) involved when choosing bypass surgery. And a disappointing number of people will not return to work afterward. Some patients are seemingly incapacitated and never regain their preoperative level of activity.

We cannot know in advance the answers to these questions for any given individual. We must be realistic in our patient selection, and we must be honest about the realistic benefits expected from bypass surgery.

We can draw the following conclusions about coronary artery bypass surgery:

1. Coronary bypass surgery will statistically prolong survival in select groups of patients (such as those with three-vessel disease and extremely abnormal exercise test results). However, for many, such as those with one- or two-vessel disease, survival will not be prolonged. The majority of

patients who undergo bypass surgery in the United States have not had their lives saved.

2. Bypass surgery does not prevent heart attacks.

3. Bypass surgery is extremely effective in relieving symptoms of angina. However, many patients slowly develop recurrent symptoms because of closure of grafts and progression of disease in the native coronary arteries.

4. Some patients will eventually require a second (and possibly a third) operation. The surgery cannot be considered a permanent solution, but on average a ten-year repair.

Balloon Angioplasty

In September 1977 a new procedure was introduced. Called balloon angioplasty (technically known as Percutaneous Transluminal Coronary Angioplasty, or PTCA), it was found to be capable of fixing the arteries of the heart. The use of balloon angioplasty has rapidly expanded over the past decade, and it is expected that more than 150,000 procedures will be performed each year in this country alone. With the increased volume has come greater public awareness, great public expectations, and many myths.

Angioplasty is a relatively simple procedure. A cardiac catheterization is performed. After a blockage is identified in a coronary artery, a small wire is advanced forward. A collapsed balloon, wrapped around the wire, is pushed into the middle of the blockage. It is then inflated, forcing the blockage open.

The artery is stretched and the cholesterol plaque is pulverized by the procedure. The artery is opened for normal blood flow.

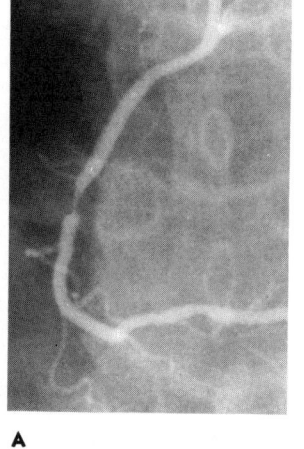
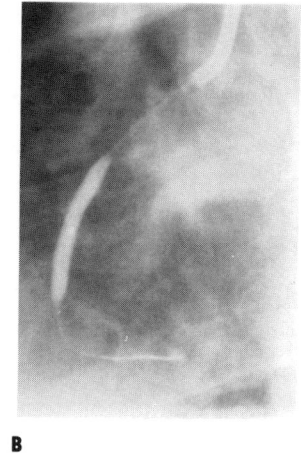
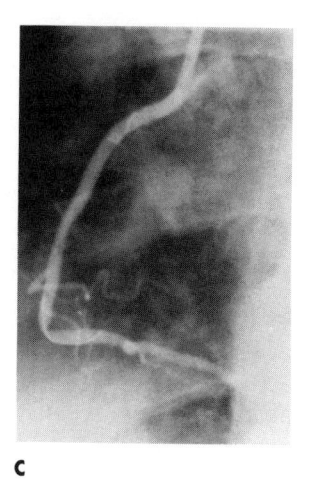

A   B   C

Balloon Angioplasty
A. Injecting contrast material reveals a 95% blockage.
B. Collapsed balloon is inserted and inflated. (No contrast material is injected, and thus only inflated balloon is visible.)
C. The blockage has been eliminated.

Surgery is not required, and only local anesthesia is used, so the patient can go home after three days in the hospital. This has made the procedure an attractive alternative to surgery.

Myth #9:
Angioplasty should replace bypass surgery in all patients.

Frank B., a sixty-two-year-old man who suffered a heart attack, had an angiogram revealing three blocked arteries. Surgery was recommended, but he requested that the balloon be used to fix his heart.

Many people, like Frank, would choose balloon angioplasty over a more invasive bypass operation. However, there are certain limitations to angioplasty that should be considered:

1. *There are risks involved in angioplasty*. For a simple repair of one artery, there is a 0.5 percent to 1.0 percent chance of death, 2 percent to 3 percent chance of having a heart attack, and a 2 percent to 3 percent chance of a bypass operation being required. The risk of the procedure increases if more than one artery is repaired. Frank could face up to a 2 percent to 3 percent chance of death for an angioplasty effort of all three blocked arteries (which is slightly greater than the risk of death from a bypass operation).

2. *Angioplasty does not always work forever*. Up to 30 percent of all arteries that are repaired will re-narrow (called "re-stenosis") within six months of angioplasty, requiring a second or a third effort. We do not understand why re-stenosis occurs, although it is suspected that the artery partially collapses where it had been stretched by the balloon.

> Nina K., a fifty-two-year-old woman, had a balloon angioplasty with a "perfect" result. She did well, until four months later, when she developed recurrent episodes of chest pain. An angiogram revealed that her artery had renarrowed.

Some arteries will fail to remain repaired, even after multiple angioplasties. The patient may then require a bypass operation. The good news is that if the artery does *not* re-stenose within six months, it has only a 1 percent-per-year re-stenosis rate thereafter.

3. *Angioplasty has* not *been demonstrated to save lives*. Whereas bypass surgery has been demonstrated to improve

survival in select patients, it is not known whether this applies for balloon angioplasty. Scientists are now involved in comparing the two techniques, and the results will be available in several years. Currently, angioplasty is known to be effective only for the relief of symptoms.

Bill M., a forty-five-year-old man who felt "completely healthy," had an exercise test before entering a health club. Because the test had a surprisingly abnormal result, he had an angiogram, which revealed an 80 percent blockage in one of his coronary arteries. His doctor recommended angioplasty.

Because Bill has no symptoms, angioplasty can't make him feel better. (It cannot relieve symptoms that are not there.) And angioplasty is not known to offer an improvement in long-term health. Without further data, for all we know, the procedure may be as likely to cause a heart attack as it is to prevent one. As a result, there is no currently accepted indication to dilate an artery in a patient who, like Bill, has no symptoms.

Although angioplasty is attractive and often effective, it is not a *replacement* for bypass surgery. It is a reasonable procedure for the relief of symptoms in patients with one- and two-vessel disease. For patients with more extensive disease, its role is currently unclear.

New modifications are being tested to improve the safety and long-term efficacy of angioplasty. These include the use of lasers, "atherectomy" catheters (which scoop out the cholesterol), and mechanical coils (called stents), which hold the artery open after the balloon dilation. It is currently unknown whether these modifications will be successful.

CHAPTER FOUR

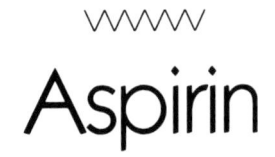

Aspirin

Aspirin is difficult to consider seriously. We are so accustomed to it in our day-to-day lives that many of us are unaware of its potency. We commonly take aspirin to lower our temperature (when we have a fever) and to relieve minor aches and pains. But we rarely expect it to do anything important. It just seems too ordinary.

Aspirin, however, has many effects on the body. It is perhaps the most effective drug available for preventing heart attacks. Aspirin is further given to almost all people who have had coronary bypass surgery in order to keep the grafts open. With a growing impact on the practice of cardiac medicine, it is even being called a "wonder drug."

But aspirin also has a dark side. It can be responsible for serious and even life-threatening bleeding problems, including bleeding into the brain. In children it has been linked to a fatal condition called Reye's syndrome. And aspirin is the most common cause of fatal drug overdose in children (it is available in most households, and parents are often unaware of its dangers).

Some people confuse aspirin and Tylenol. They are very different (Tylenol has no effect on the heart). And even more people are confused about what they should do as individuals. Should everyone be taking aspirin? What dose (adult or baby) should be taken? And how often?

Myth #1:
Aspirin is not a drug.

Because aspirin is available over the counter, it is not viewed as a very serious drug. But had it been invented today, aspirin would have a difficult time becoming approved by the Food and Drug Administration, and might even have been classified a prescription drug.

But aspirin beat the system by being around for a long time. For more than 1,000 years the Chinese have treated fevers using the bark of the willow tree, which contains salicin, a chemical precursor of aspirin. In the early 1800s different derivatives of this bark were discovered and tested. Acetylsalicylic acid (the chemical name for aspirin) was found to be the best tolerated. Aspirin was officially introduced in 1899, and has been marketed in its current form for more than eighty years.

Because it was already available when the FDA was created, aspirin was permitted (by a grandfather clause) to remain an over-the-counter medication, and was thus not subjected to the same scrutiny that *new* medicines currently receive.

What Does Aspirin Do?

Aspirin interferes with the production of a series of chemicals in our bodies called prostaglandins. This family of chemicals regulates many of our body's vital functions. There are different types of prostaglandins in different parts of the body. Aspirin blocks the production of some prostaglandins, affecting the response of the body in many different situations.

Some of these effects are very useful, while others are potentially harmful. The major effects of taking an aspirin include:

1. *Lowering temperature.* Prostaglandins raise the temperature of the body. Aspirin, by blocking these prostaglandins, will lower it.

2. *Relieving minor aches and pains, including headache.* Prostaglandins contribute to the brain's awareness of pain. Aspirin blocks this awareness.

3. *Relieving inflammation.* Prostaglandins play a major role in creating inflammation in the body. Aspirin is very effective at reducing this response. Arthritis is defined as inflammation of the joints, and aspirin is remarkably effective in treating this condition.

4. *Interfering with blood clotting.* This is the big one for heart disease. Prostaglandins play a major role in blood clotting. Aspirin is helpful for patients with heart disease because it blocks this effect, causing a "thinning" of the blood. But this also is why aspirin is dangerous.

The last two actions of aspirin are clinically the most important. The ability of aspirin to reduce inflammation is dramatic. In fact, aspirin is the standard of comparison for a series of prescription drugs available for the relief of inflammation (such as Motrin, Indocin, Naprosyn, Feldene, and Voltarin). These "aspirinlike" drugs block prostaglandins, and are widely used in the United States for the relief of arthritis pain.

But aspirin is the most potent of them all. It will relieve arthritis pain as well as, or better than, any of those in the competition (which are also more expensive). But it has some important disadvantages.

Aspirin must be taken five to six times a day to achieve its optimal effect, whereas the others drugs will be effective when taken only once or twice a day. The high dose of aspirin required to relieve pain is often associated with bad side effects, which include ringing in the ears, fatigue, stomach irritation and ulcers, and possibly internal bleeding. Some people are unable to tolerate aspirin and must use the less-toxic (and perhaps less-effective) alternative drugs.

The ability of aspirin to interfere with blood clotting has made it an invaluable drug in modern cardiology. The other drugs have only a very weak effect, and are not used in treating heart disease.

Myth #2:
Aspirin and Tylenol are the same thing.

Aspirin and Tylenol are *not* the same thing. Although they are both used to reduce fever and relieve minor pain, aspirin is a much more diverse drug. Tylenol (acetaminophen is the chemical name) does not inhibit the production of prostaglandins. It has a different chemical effect in the brain, lowering temperature and relieving pain. Although these results are similar to those of aspirin, they occur through a different mechanism.

Because Tylenol has no effect on prostaglandin, it does not reduce inflammation and it does not interfere with blood clotting. Therefore, Tylenol is not useful in treating heart disease (and it is not very effective in treating arthritis).

The aspirinlike drugs, mentioned earlier, partially interfere with prostaglandin, making them similar to aspirin, but not the same. They are effective at reducing inflammation, and hence are excellent medicines for treating arthritis. They relieve headache and can even lower temperature. But they do not have a big effect on blood clotting, and therefore are not very good for treating heart disease.

Comparing aspirin, Tylenol, and Motrin (as a representative of the aspirinlike drugs), examine the following chart:

ACTION OF DRUGS

DRUG	PAIN	TEMPERATURE	INFLAMMATION	BLOOD CLOTTING
Aspirin	+ +	+ + + +	+ + +	+ + +
Tylenol	+ +	+ + + +	none	none
Motrin	+ +	+ + +	+ + +	+

+ + + Strongly effective + + Moderately effective + Mildly effective

Aspirin is the drug that is the most effective in inhibiting blood clotting. We sometimes refer to aspirin as a "blood thinner." Tylenol has *no* effect, whereas Motrin (and the other related drugs) has a minor effect on blood clotting.

Myth #3:
Aspirin will literally "thin" the blood.

The term "blood thinner" is more metaphoric than literal. The blood will not be any less viscous after a person takes an aspirin, and it will appear completely normal in a test tube. However, it will take longer for bleeding to stop after aspirin because of the effect it has on platelets, a key component of blood clotting.

Platelets are tiny cellular fragments that act as a natural "sticky" substance in the blood. Their normal role is to initiate blood clotting. They are the first defense against bleeding. But they are not very "intelligent." They are the most simple of all the components of the blood. The platelets will stick to anything if they are stimulated. Usually, it takes an injury to a blood vessel to stimulate the platelets.

The platelets travel through the circulatory system just waiting to stick to something. They constantly look for a hole or tear in a blood vessel. When they find one, they clump together (by the millions), forming a plug in the hole.

Initially the plug is weak, and the repair is temporary. But as they start to stick together, the platelets call for help. They send out chemicals that activate the blood-clotting factors. A blood clot forms, which is a much stronger repair.

This system can backfire. For unknown reasons, the platelets sometimes begin to clump together in places where they should not, leading to inappropriate clot formation. When it happens in an artery supplying the heart muscle with blood, a heart attack occurs.

Without prostaglandins, platelets would not stick together. Aspirin chemically wipes out the ability of platelets to make prostaglandin, making them no longer sticky. One adult aspirin will permanently inactivate all of the platelets in the blood (and there are millions of them!). In fact, only a fraction of an adult aspirin (only one-tenth) is required to inactivate all of the platelets in the circulation.

But platelets are constantly replenished by the bone marrow (the "factory" that makes all of the cells of the blood). Platelets usually last only ten to fourteen days in the circulation. Every day, therefore, approximately 10 percent of our platelets are normally turned over. The newly released platelets are not affected by a dose of aspirin given the day before. They will work normally, unless a new aspirin is given that day.

Doctors usually request that a patient *not* take any aspirin for at least a week before elective surgery. One aspirin taken close to the time of the operation will result in more intra-operative bleeding and an increased likelihood of the patient needing a blood transfusion. Waiting one week after the last dose of aspirin allows enough normal platelets to accumulate in the circulation to permit normal blood clotting.

Taking one aspirin every day will inactivate the new plate-lets after they are released into the circulation. Therefore, blood clotting remains inhibited. This is very good for the heart.

Why Is It Good to "Thin" the Blood?

Heart attacks are caused by the sudden, catastrophic, and complete blockage of blood flow in one of the three arteries of the heart. If flow through one of these coronary arteries is abruptly interrupted, a section of heart muscle will stop work-ing and eventually die.

More than 95 percent of heart attacks are precipitated by a blood clot. There is usually a preexisting narrowing (due to cholesterol) in the artery, that has developed over many years. For reasons not fully understood, the cholesterol block-age can suddenly undergo a change, causing it to attract platelets to stick on its surface. This results in the formation of a blood clot, which blocks the artery and causes a heart attack.

Platelet activation is an important step in this process. Aspirin blocks the activation of platelets and thereby lowers the likelihood of a heart attack occurring.

Myth #4:
If one aspirin can prevent blood clotting, more must be better.

Peter J., a seventy-two-year-old man with heart disease, has been placed on two different heart medications (each to be taken three times a day). In addition, his doctor recommended that one adult aspirin be taken every morning. Peter decided that more must be better, and decided to take two aspirin every time he took his other heart medicines (a total of six aspirin a day).

One month later, Peter began to notice some mild stomach pains. He awoke one night nauseated, and he vomited a small amount of blood. In the emergency room he was discovered to be anemic. The aspirin had irritated his stomach, causing it to bleed. Peter required a transfusion of two units of blood.

Aspirin is a stomach irritant. It can cause erosions, ulcers, and irritation (called gastritis), all of which can result in internal bleeding. Aspirin delivers a one-two punch because it *also* inhibits blood clotting. When stomach bleeding occurs, it is less easily controlled by the body.

The destructive effects on the stomach are directly related to the dose of aspirin. One aspirin a day is much less likely to cause gastric bleeding than six aspirin a day. Taking more aspirin significantly increases the chances of bleeding. It is a common myth that either buffered or coated aspirin absolutely prevent gastric bleeding. The long-term use of these products, especially in large doses, carries the same risk of complications as taking regular aspirin.

A single adult aspirin (325 milligrams in strength) will block all of the platelets in the circulation. But this is pharmacologic overkill. Only 40 milligrams of aspirin are required to do the same thing. A "baby" aspirin (which is 80 milligrams) is therefore effective when given to patients with heart disease. It has twice the strength required to block all the platelets, yet it is much less likely (because of its low strength) to irritate the stomach.

Many patients are surprised when a baby aspirin is recommended. It is difficult to think of an orange-flavored, chewable aspirin for children as a real drug. But it is a real drug, and has very real effects on the body.

Less aspirin is less toxic. This is a good reason to avoid large doses. But less aspirin may actually be *better* for the heart than larger doses. This is because of a fascinating chemical balance in the heart.

The inhibition of the prostaglandins found in platelets is a "good" effect. But other prostaglandins in the body are blocked by aspirin, which is not always desirable. One such prostaglandin is responsible for dilating the coronary arteries (which are the fuel lines on the surface of the heart). Blocking these prostaglandins with aspirin will block this desirable effect. Fortunately, the prostaglandins in the coronary arteries are *less sensitive* to the effects of aspirin, and will not be blocked by doses under 325 milligrams (an adult pill).

It is best to give the smallest dose of aspirin possible. Extra aspirin, above one pill each day, can counteract the effect of blocking platelets by further blocking the important natural dilator of the coronary arteries.

Some scientists have suggested that the optimal dose may be only 40 milligrams (half a baby aspirin). This dose will block platelets, have no effect on the coronary arteries, and will have minimal toxicity. This low dose has not been proven effective in scientific studies, but it is under consideration. However, it is certain that more is *not* better.

Myth #5:
An aspirin will prevent heart attacks in everyone.

Although this is not true, it has been the focus of much attention by scientists, the media, and the public. There is a great deal of theoretical information that suggests aspirin would be good for widespread use. Aspirin is already called a wonder drug. But who should actually be taking aspirin? Should it be given only to people with diagnosed (and therefore known) heart disease? Or should everybody, including healthy adults, take aspirin every day?

There have been a fair number of studies addressing the issue of who will benefit from aspirin. The majority tested aspirin in people who *already had* heart disease, and aspirin was very successful. Only two studies examined aspirin in otherwise healthy people, and they had mixed results.

We will first explore the impact of aspirin on people with different forms of heart disease: unstable angina, heart attack, and after bypass surgery. Afterward, we will consider the general public.

Unstable Angina

Impressive results were obtained in the Veterans Administration study of aspirin given to people with unstable angina.[1] This heart condition is characterized by progressively worsening episodes of chest pain, often resulting in a heart attack. The activation of the blood-clotting system plays an important role in this process.

While heart attacks are caused by the total obstruction of

an artery supplying the heart, in unstable angina the coronary artery is only partially occluded by a blood clot. The clot grows in size, causing unstable symptoms as the artery becomes progressively narrowed.

The Veterans Administration study enrolled more than 1,200 men with unstable angina, and followed them for a twelve-week period. The men were treated equally, except that half were given one adult aspirin (325 milligrams) every day. The other half received a placebo pill, which looked like the aspirin. Otherwise, the men received exactly the same medical care. Yet there was a dramatic difference in outcome.

There was a 50 percent reduction in the number of cardiac events in the group treated with aspirin. Among the men given the placebo, 10 percent either died or had a heart attack. In contrast, only 5 percent among the men treated with aspirin had a cardiac event.

This ordinary medicine saved lives, and taking one aspirin each day was relatively safe, easy, and inexpensive. As a result, aspirin has become a standard medication in the treatment of unstable angina.

Patients Who Have Survived Heart Attacks

Aspirin also will help those who have had a heart attack. Six different large-scale scientific studies, collectively involving more than 10,000 such patients, have demonstrated that taking aspirin can be very important.[2]

Many heart attack survivors will continue to have heart problems *after* they go home, especially during the first year of recovery. In the different studies those taking aspirin had, on average, a 10 percent reduction in the likelihood of death and a 20 percent reduction in the occurrence of second heart attacks. Thus aspirin is now a standard part of the medication list after hospital discharge.

Patients in the Midst
of a Heart Attack

A study from Europe has further suggested that aspirin can be helpful if given immediately during a heart attack.

The study, called ISIS (International Study of Infarct Survival) involved more than 17,000 people enrolled during the first twenty-four hours of a heart attack.[3] Half of these patients were immediately given one adult aspirin, while the other half received a placebo pill. The treatment was otherwise the same for the two groups, but the difference in outcome was impressive.

Taking aspirin lowered the number of people who died from their heart attacks. Whereas 11.8 percent of people died in the hospital when given the placebo pill, only 9.4 percent died when given a single aspirin daily. This is a reduction in the total mortality of 2.6 percent.

Each year in the United States more than 700,000 people are hospitalized with heart attacks. If each of these patients were immediately given an aspirin, up to 18,000 lives could be saved. This is dramatic, especially when considering that the benefit comes from only one aspirin.

Bypass Operations

Aspirin is also very important for patients who have had coronary-artery bypass surgery. The new tubes placed in the heart unfortunately do not last forever. Up to 20 percent will develop clots and totally obstruct during the first postoperative year, and more than 50 percent will be closed by ten years after surgery. In multiple studies, aspirin has been demonstrated to reduce by 50 percent the number of grafts that will get into trouble.[4] As a result of this significant benefit, nearly all patients are given aspirin after bypass surgery. The usual dose is one adult aspirin (325 milligrams) per day, but doses as low as 100 milligrams daily have been shown to be effective in protecting bypass grafts.

There is plenty of data available to demonstrate that aspirin helps people who have heart disease (particularly those with unstable angina and heart attacks), and it has been shown that those who have had a bypass operation will do better if they take aspirin.

But it has been suggested that everyone might benefit from aspirin. There are nearly 6 million Americans with diagnosed heart disease. But there are many more adults without heart disease. Should they be taking an aspirin?

Healthy People *Without* Heart Disease

This particular issue was addressed in a well-publicized study from Harvard University called the Physicians' Health Study.[5] It is a singular study in that only healthy doctors were allowed to enter as subjects. Doctors were selected because they are easy to locate and tend to take the medicines prescribed.

A single dose of adult aspirin (325 milligrams) was given every other day to 11,037 physicians, while an additional 11,034 received a placebo pill. All the subjects were healthy and free of heart disease at the beginning of the study. In contrast, all the previous aspirin studies involved patients who had already had heart trouble.

Among the physicians receiving the placebo, there were 189 heart attacks (1.7 percent of the group) during the five years that they were followed. The group taking aspirin, on the other hand, experienced only 104 heart attacks (0.9 percent). This is a reduction of 84 heart attacks (out of 11,000 subjects) attributable to aspirin. But, not all heart attacks are fatal. In fact, aspirin did *not* save lives. The total number of cardiovascular deaths was 44 in both groups.

This is not a spectacular result. And there was even some discouraging news. A small increase in the number of strokes developed among those taking aspirin (80 strokes) compared with those on the placebo (70 strokes). Aspirin, by "thinning" the blood, made bleeding in the brain more likely.

Doctors may take better care of themselves than the general public. It is uncertain if the results of this study can be applied to patients in the "real world." A similar study, involving British doctors, found that 500 milligrams of aspirin taken every day did *not* prevent death or heart attacks, further discouraging the notion that aspirin will help everyone.[6]

It is not known whether all of us should take aspirin. Certainly those with heart disease will benefit (aspirin prevents from 10 percent to 50 percent of subsequent cardiac events). But the data are more vague when aspirin is given to healthy people.

Based on the current studies, if the entire public were to take one aspirin a day, only an extremely small number of heart attacks would be prevented. Total mortality would probably remain the same, while more bleeding and more strokes would occur. Very few people would be affected either way. For most, aspirin would do *nothing*.

Myth #6:
Aspirin may help the heart, but it is otherwise harmless.

This myth can lead to disaster. Most people do not realize that an aspirin overdose can be lethal. In fact, taking as few as thirty aspirin tablets all at once has proven to be fatal for some adults, who were performing a "suicide gesture."

Aspirin toxicity occurs as a function of dose. The earliest symptoms are dizziness, ringing in the ears, and impairment of hearing. With higher doses come nausea, vomiting, sweating, diarrhea, and drowsiness. Ultimately, aspirin intoxication is characterized by confusion, convulsions, coma, and, finally, death. These later symptoms usually require more massive doses.

Patients who take aspirin for arthritis (up to twelve to fifteen pills per day) commonly experience ringing in the ears. This early sign of toxicity indicates that the aspirin dose should be reduced.

In addition, aspirin can cause bleeding, which is somewhat independent of the dose. The effect on platelets (caused by one aspirin) results in a sluggish ability to form blood clots. In some people this can contribute to significant bleeding, possibly into the brain. Those patients on Coumadin (an extremely potent blood thinner) and those with inherited clotting problems, like hemophiliacs, must absolutely avoid aspirin.

Aspirin must be used with great care in children. In comparison with adults, much smaller doses will be fatal to a child. And yet aspirin is quite accessible in many households, making it the leading cause of drug overdose among children.

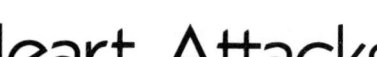

Heart Attacks

Every twenty seconds someone in the United States has a heart attack. That's more than 1.5 million every year. Only half of these people will be hospitalized. Five hundred thousand will die, most before ever reaching a hospital. Many others will fail to seek medical attention, denying there is a problem.

But there *is* a problem. Ignorance contributes to unnecessary deaths. Although we can't save everyone in the midst of a heart attack, some cardiac deaths can be prevented with proper medical care. And despite significant media attention, there remain many myths and misconceptions about heart attacks.

In recent years there has been an explosive amount of information concerning heart attacks published within the scientific world. Much of this has filtered to the public, often with an incomplete and distorted perspective, contributing to some of the confusion. Aspirin, "clot busting" drugs, emergency bypass surgery, and balloon angioplasty have all made headlines as therapies for acute heart attacks. Yet most people have only a vague idea of what happens during a heart attack, and do not understand why these various approaches are potentially valuable.

Some people know that a heart attack involves a "blockage" of blood flow, while others are aware that heart attacks have "something to do with blood clots." And still others say:

> ". . . there is a spasm."
> ". . . the heart stops beating and you die."
> ". . . there is severe pain in the chest."
> ". . . the heart is attacked."

There is a little bit of truth in each of these statements. But they are all vague. Heart attacks are very different events for different people. There are few myths here, because most people haven't a clear idea of what a heart attack is in the first place. But the definition is straightforward: *a heart attack is the death of some amount of heart muscle.*

This is simple and exact. A heart attack involves the death of some amount of heart muscle, whether it be a large or small amount, and whether it comes from the right or left side of the heart.

The heart is divided into two main muscular pumps, called the ventricles.

The first pump (the right ventricle) receives blood from the veins of the body, and then ejects it into the lungs. The blood mixes with the air we breathe, receiving oxygen. The now oxygen-rich blood enters the next pump (the left ventricle), where it is ejected into the aorta. The blood is sent through the aorta and its many branches to the entire body, to be used as fuel.

The left ventricle is the more important pump because it

is responsible for pushing blood into the main circulation. Damage to the left ventricle is therefore crucial during heart attacks. Damage to the right ventricle is more easily tolerated.

The left ventricle has five major walls of muscle, all of which contribute to the pumping action: bottom (inferior), front (anterior), back (posterior), and two side walls (septal and lateral).

These walls are not anatomically distinct; they blend into one another. When the left ventricle is stimulated to contract, they all squeeze down, and together they push blood out of the heart. When any amount of this muscle dies (involving any or all of the walls), it is called a heart attack.

Why does heart muscle die?

It dies because it is deprived of oxygen and nutrients. All living things require fuel to stay alive. This fuel is delivered by blood.

Some organs are more sensitive to the loss of fuel and will die more quickly than others. The cells of the brain will die within minutes of losing blood flow. On the other hand, the arms and legs can last for hours. The heart, which is the source of fuel to the rest of the body, also requires fuel to survive. The muscle of the heart is like all other living things. It must receive fresh blood to work and to stay alive.

Ironically, the left ventricle (the main pumping chamber of the heart) is filled with the oxygen-rich blood it needs to survive. But the heart can't simply suck the blood out of this chamber. If it could, there would never be heart attacks. Instead, the blood must first be pumped out of the left ventricle and ejected into the aorta (the main fuel line of the entire body).

From the aorta, blood is distributed through smaller arteries to every part of the body. There are arteries that carry blood to the brain (cerebral arteries), to the stomach (gastric arteries), and to the kidneys (renal arteries). Some of the blood returns to the heart muscle through three special branches called the "coronary arteries."

The three coronary arteries run on the outside surface of the heart. They further divide into smaller branches that penetrate into the heart muscle and deliver blood and oxygen to every cell of the heart. This is how the heart gets its fuel. Fresh, oxygen-rich blood must be ejected out of the heart's pumping chamber before it can return fuel the muscle itself.

We have defined "heart attack" as the death of heart muscle. We can now expand this definition. The heart muscle dies *because* it is deprived of fuel. Further, it is deprived of fuel as one of the fuel lines to the heart (the coronary arteries) becomes obstructed. This is the complete definition of a heart attack.

Three Coronary Arteries

There are three arteries that supply the heart with blood. Each artery acts like a river, delivering blood to the different sections of the muscle of the heart. One of the three arteries supplies the right side of the heart; it's aptly named the right coronary artery (RCA). The other two arteries supply the left side of the heart; they are the left anterior descending (LAD) artery and the circumflex artery (CIRC).

Each of the five walls of the left ventricle is supplied by branches from these three arteries. In most people the RCA supplies the bottom wall (inferior), the LAD supplies the front wall (anterior) and one of the side walls (septal), and the CIRC supplies the back wall (posterior) and the other side wall (lateral).

These arteries can't usually help one another out, because

there is virtually no overlap in the territories that they supply. When one artery becomes blocked, the other arteries can't bring relief blood to the area that is in need.

For example, if the LAD artery were totally occluded, the front and side walls of the left ventricle would suddenly be deprived of all blood flow. The RCA and CIRC would be unable to send extra blood to the rescue because they do not send branches to these walls. These sections of heart muscle would die without fresh blood, and the patient would experience a heart attack (in this case, a large one).

There are some exceptions. Some fortunate people have arteries that actually can help one another. They have developed microscopic channels that link the different arteries. These channels are called "collaterals." If one artery becomes occluded, the other arteries can send blood to the deprived heart muscle through these tiny collaterals, potentially preventing the death of the muscle.

People are not born with these collaterals; it is not known why some people develop them and others do not. One possibility is that arteries, with long-standing blockages (from atherosclerosis), may produce a chemical that stimulates the slow growth of these collaterals. This chemical has not been identified.

It is possible that only some of us have the ability to make this chemical, while others do not. Also, it may take many years to "grow" the collaterals even with the necessary chemical stimulation.

We do not know the answers to many of these mysteries, but there is great scientific interest in identifying the chemical(s) that stimulate collateral growth. It is hoped that one day we may develop a medicine capable of creating these protective channels in more heart patients.

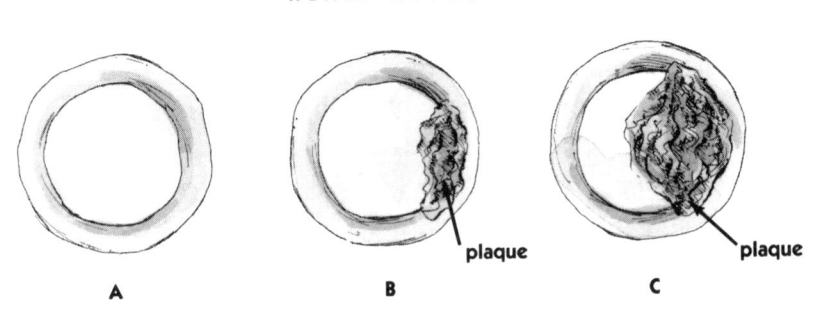

Growing Plaque in Arteries
Seen here in cross-section, cholesterol deposits in the wall of an artery
may accumulate over many years: A. Normal; B. Mild blockage five
years later; C. Much greater blockage ten years later.

What Blocks the
Arteries During Heart Attacks?

It is easy to become confused when we discuss a "blocked"
artery. Atherosclerosis (also called plaque, or even hardening
of the arteries) causes arteries to be narrowed and blocked.
Blood clots also cause arteries to be blocked. Which is responsible for causing a heart attack?

In fact, it is a combination of both. Atherosclerosis is a
slow, chronic condition that creates long-standing narrowings
in the arteries of the heart. This sets the stage for the formation
of a blood clot, which is responsible for completely occluding
the coronary artery and causing a heart attack. The formation
of a blood clot within an artery is sudden and catastrophic.

Cholesterol, fat, cellular debris, and calcium all deposit
inside the walls of coronary arteries, creating atherosclerotic
plaque. These plaques grow slowly in size over the years,
clogging the fuel lines and thereby limiting blood flow.

—

This process is the so-called hardening of the arteries. We commonly measure the narrowing caused by a plaque as the percentage of the diameter of the artery that is blocked.

A normal artery, without any blockage, permits a surplus of blood to travel to the heart muscle. As a result, an artery is not considered to be significantly narrowed unless the plaque obstructs more than 50 percent of the artery's diameter. Even when the artery is 50 percent occluded, enough blood can reach the heart to allow it to work normally.

Patients with insignificant blockages (50 percent or less) are usually without symptoms. They would be expected to have a normal checkup in the doctor's office (including having a normal result on a stress test). Once the blockage exceeds 50 percent, however, important reductions of blood flow begin to occur. The patient might experience symptoms (chest pain with activity) and have abnormal results on testing.

A blockage of 90 percent significantly limits the amount of fuel reaching the heart muscle. Such a narrowing would limit the activity of the heart, preventing it from performing extra work. But even with a 90 percent blockage, enough blood can pass through the artery to keep the heart muscle alive. Heart muscle will remain alive even when there is a 99 percent blockage in its fuel line.

Heart attacks will not occur until a blockage becomes total. Heart muscle does not die until there is obstruction of *all* blood flow through the artery. And complete obstruction will occur only when a blood clot forms abruptly, blocking all blood flow downstream. But it is almost always a combination of a clot (acute) and a plaque (chronic) that results in this medical disaster.

Blood clots do not (usually) form on the surface of a normal artery. The body will prevent this. Even the somewhat irregular surface of atherosclerotic plaque resists the formation of a blood clot. In most people plaques grow for years without causing any problems. However, for reasons not fully understood, the plaque's surface can change abruptly and encourage the formation of a blood clot, resulting in a heart attack.

This appears to be the result of a physical change in the plaque itself. Its surface literally cracks giving the body the false signal that it needs to form a blood clot. A clot thus forms, totally occluding the artery.

Sometimes the body's clotting system is the culprit causing a clot to form even if the plaque does not change. Different types of stress can inappropriately activate the clotting system, leading to clot formation in previously stable parts of the body.

The following example demonstrates how a clot can form in an artery that has a minimal blockage, because of a super-activated clotting system.

Lisa B., a thirty-eight-year-old woman who came to the hospital with severe chest pain, was found to be experiencing a moderately large heart attack. Lisa was, at the time, taking birth-control pills and smoking two packs of cigarettes a day. In the emergency room she received one of the new "clot-busting" drugs, which successfully dissolved the clot and restored blood flow to the heart muscle.

Three days later an angiogram revealed a 40 percent narrowing of one of the three arteries supplying her heart. The other two coronary arteries were totally normal, without any blockages. Lisa had no further symptoms.

Prior to going home (eight days after the heart attack) she had a normal exercise stress test. Lisa stopped taking her birth-control pills and quit smoking.

Lisa experienced a heart attack because a blood clot formed in one of her coronary arteries. Although the underlying atherosclerosis obstructed only 40 percent of the artery, the sudden addition of a blood clot resulted in complete occlusion. The clot filled in the remaining 60 percent of the artery.

This is unusual. Although young people can have minimal atherosclerotic disease (usually under 50 percent), they usually do *not* have heart attacks. But, in this case, a clot formed because Lisa's blood had been made excessively "sticky" by her cigarette smoking and by her use of birth-control pills.

Cigarette smoking activates platelets, and birth-control pills activate many of the clotting factors in the blood. The combination of the two is notorious for creating excessive blood clotting, leading to premature heart attacks, strokes, and fatal blood clots to the lungs (pulmonary embolism).

Young women like Lisa who both smoke and take oral contraceptives are at high risk for these disasters (even at very young ages). This explains why a clot can form in an artery that is only 40 percent narrowed.

Cigarette smoking, even without the addition of birth-control pills, makes the blood very sticky. This is one reason why smokers have more heart attacks than non-smokers.

Cocaine also causes activation of the blood-clotting system, and has been responsible for heart attacks occurring in very young people. The use of cocaine has caused clots to form even in completely normal coronary arteries. This is extraordinary, because clots usually require some plaque to latch onto. But cocaine is a powerful stimulant, making the blood sticky enough to form a clot, with or without underlying atherosclerotic disease.

Fortunately, the blood usually returns to normal after the removal of these substances, and the risk of experiencing a premature heart attack is significantly reduced. On the other hand, continuing to smoke, use cocaine, or take the Pill further activates blood clotting and increases the risk of heart attacks and strokes.

There is a balance between the role of the underlying atherosclerotic plaque and the degree of stickiness of the blood. Very sticky blood can cause clots to form in an artery with little plaque, while a severely narrowed artery may not require quite as much blood stickiness to form a clot. If the surface of a plaque ruptures, regardless of its size, a clot may form.

When a patient arrives in an emergency room with a heart attack, one can't immediataely tell what percentage of the complete coronary artery occlusion is blood clot and what percentage is atherosclerosis. We know that the artery is 100 percent blocked, by some combination of the two.

When Lisa came to the emergency room, 40 percent of her artery was obstructed by atherosclerosis. Thus, the remaining 60 percent of her artery was blocked by a blood clot. A different patient might have a heart attack with an artery blocked 90 percent by plaque and only 10 percent by a clot. In both examples the end result is the total blockage of the artery.

Regardless of the cause of the occlusion of an artery, the amount of muscle that dies is more important.

The Size of the Heart Attack

The size of a heart attack depends on the size of the artery that is blocked. Bigger arteries have a greater amount of heart muscle depending on them. If a large artery becomes totally blocked, large amounts of heart muscle may die. Conversely, if only a small artery becomes occluded, there will be less damage. Sometimes only a branch of an artery becomes occluded, usually resulting in a heart attack of limited size.

The front (anterior) wall, supplied by the LAD, is the largest and most important of the five walls. Damage here has the greatest impact on the net strength of the heart, and front-wall heart attacks are usually the most severe. The total amount of muscle that is damaged during a heart attack is of prime importance.

The loss of 40 percent of the muscle of the left ventricle usually results in the death of the patient because the heart is too weak to keep the body alive. In contrast, some heart attacks are so small (very little muscle dies) that the overall function of the heart is not diminished. But big or small, a heart attack means that some amount of muscle dies.

The heart has a job to do. It must continually deliver enough fuel to meet the demands of the body, or the body will die. When we are physically active, our bodies require more fuel than when we are sitting in a chair. Hence, the heart must work faster and harder to meet the body's greater demands during intense activity.

The heart has large amounts of reserve strength and it will usually compensate for mild to moderate amounts of damage. When one wall is damaged, the other walls will work harder, allowing the heart to continue to deliver enough fuel to meet the needs of the body. But if a heart attack is very large, compensation becomes more difficult.

With greater amounts of damage, the remaining heart muscle will not be enough to compensate for the loss. The heart becomes incapable of delivering enough blood for the body to perform its job normally. This results in crises in other organs of the body, which is called shock. There is not enough fuel delivered for the kidneys, liver, and brain to stay alive.

Each year in the United States 750,000 people are admitted to hospitals with heart attacks (big or small). Those with small heart attacks have a 3 percent chance of dying before going home, while those with moderate to large heart attacks have anywhere from a 15 percent to 60 percent mortality. The death rate is greater than 95 percent for those who experience massive heart attacks that are complicated by shock.

We do not have the technology available to measure directly and accurately the amount of heart muscle that dies during a heart attack. How, then, can we tell if a heart attack has been small or large? We tell by measuring the overall strength of the *surviving* heart muscle (which is easy to do). If a heart attack has been large, then the surviving heart muscle will be proportionately weak.

Measuring the Strength of the Heart: The Ejection Fraction

We measure the strength of the heart by counting how much blood is squeezed out with each beat. Before beating, the left ventricle fills with blood. The five walls then squeeze down, pushing most (but not all) of this blood out of the pumping chamber and into the aorta. It will hold on to the remaining blood, fill up with fresh blood from the lungs, then squeeze once again.

The percentage of blood that is ejected out of the heart is called the "ejection fraction." In healthy people, relaxing comfortably, the ejection fraction is usually between 50 percent and 60 percent. With vigorous exercise, the heart must work harder. The walls of the left ventricle squeeze down with more intensity, causing a greater percentage of blood to be ejected into the circulation. The ejection fraction might increase up to 70 percent during times of exercise (if the heart is healthy). A sick heart might not be able to beat more strongly with exercise, often leading to a sense of weakness and fatigue. But even with the most strenuous exercise a healthy heart will not eject all the blood from its pumping chamber; thus, the ejection fraction never reaches 100 percent.

There are several tests that can measure the heart's ejection fraction. After a heart attack, the ejection fraction is expected to be depressed below normal because the heart has suffered damage. *The bigger the heart attack, the weaker the heart,* resulting in a lower ejection fraction and a gloomier prognosis for the patient.

Doctors observe that people with very weak hearts (with a severely depressed ejection fraction) are more likely to die suddenly than those with strong hearts. For reasons we do not fully understand, these injured hearts are more likely to stop without warning. With serious underlying damage, this is more likely to happen. In the following chapter, on "sudden death," we will explore the different ways that the heart can suddenly stop. Some are related to the muscle failing, while others to disruption of the heart's "electrical system."

If the ejection fraction is greater than 45 percent, the prognosis for the patient is excellent. If it is lower than 30 percent, the prognosis is quite poor. Reviewing the outcome of patients at The New York Hospital, survival was related to ejection fraction as follows[1]:

Ejection Fraction	Survival during 2.5 years
>45%	99%
30% to 44%	96%
<30%	46%

Some people are found to have ejection fractions as low as 15 percent to 20 percent, reflecting profound damage to the heart muscle. These people have only a 50 percent chance of surviving for one year. But these are only averages. We can't tell the future for any given patient. We can't predict with certainty who will live and who will die. We can only estimate the odds of survival.

Ralph T. was a forty-nine-year-old reporter who suffered a huge heart attack. Two weeks afterward the ejection fraction of his left ventricle was measured to be 19 percent. He was weakened from the heart attack but eventually returned to work. He found it difficult to spend an entire day at the office, and often required a nap. He lacked the strength to climb stairs, run, or even walk quickly. Although he had been relatively athletic before the heart attack, he was now greatly limited in his activity.

Ralph survived against the odds for five years, dying suddenly at work one day.

This is an uncommon example because Ralph lived longer than statistics would predict. He had not been expected to survive for more than one or two years after the heart attack. But some people will beat the averages, which is why it is not possible to tell any person how long he or she will live.

The quality of one's life is as important as one's life expectancy. Ralph discovered that he was unable to perform at his pre–heart attack level of activity. He was left feeling weak and tired, unable to exercise or to push himself as he did before his heart attack. To his credit, he returned to work. Many in his position are unable to do so.

The quality of one's life usually becomes affected when the heart is severely damaged. When the ejection fraction falls below 33 percent, the heart will begin to have trouble meeting the needs of the body, especially during times of exercise.

A person with an ejection fraction of 19 percent, such as in the example of Ralph, will pump enough blood to allow the body to perform simple activities. But the heart will not eject enough blood to permit the body to do greater amounts of work or exercise.

But even here there are exceptions.

Tom G., a fifty-three-year-old man, suffered a very large heart attack. His left ventricle was found to have an ejection fraction of 19 percent. After several months of recovery Tom returned to playing tennis (albeit less vigorously than before the heart attack), climbing stairs, and performing most activities that he wanted to. Tom defied the odds, and his doctor's advice (who felt that tennis was too much of a stress). He was more active than one would have predicted.

Obviously no single measurement or number is enough to predict everything. We have many guidelines. Although medicine is filled with exceptions, the majority of people conform to the rules.

We have discussed the heart muscle, the coronary arteries, and the definition of a heart attack. Now we will examine the common myths associated with this medical event.

Myth #1:
"If I have chest pressure, then I'm not having a heart attack. Heart attacks are painful."

Heart attacks can certainly be very painful. But many patients insist that they are feeling pressure in their chest, *not pain*. This may seem like an arbitrary difference, yet it is amazing how many people will deny having pain. When asked if they are having pressure, they will answer yes. They simply deny that the pressure is painful.

Some people delay going to the hospital, or stay home altogether, because they assume that pressure in the chest is all right. But pressure is a common symptom of a heart attack, and should be taken seriously.

Some heart attacks will cause pain (or pressure) in the arms, shoulders, back, or even jaw. This makes diagnosis difficult. Doctors must carefully consider the general nature and severity of the symptoms. The patient's age and presence of underlying cardiac risk factors (smoking, high blood pressure, diabetes) are also important. For example, we would be more concerned about chest pain in a sixty-two-year-old man who smokes cigarettes than in a fifty-eight-year-old-man who does not. Because we can't always be certain, doctors tend to be conservative and assume that any questionable symptom is emanating from the heart until it is proven otherwise.

Up to 20 percent of all heart attacks go unnoticed. Some of them are dismissed by patients as indigestion or "heartburn," while others are totally silent. A "silent heart attack" is one that occurs without manifesting any symptoms. The patients are unaware that there is a problem, and can experience sudden death without warning. These patients will not know that they have had a heart attack unless it is discovered by routine testing later on.

Silent heart attacks are more common among people with diabetes. Diabetes often causes damage to nerves throughout the body, including the nerves supplying the heart. The brain will not know the heart is in pain if the nervous system has been interrupted. Heart attacks are silent in these patients because the brain is *unaware* of the painful problem.

Myth #2:
Severe chest pain is always a heart attack.

Carl O., a forty-eight-year-old man admitted to the hospital with severe chest pain, stated that he had suffered from three "heart attacks" in the past five years. Yet his medical records revealed that he had never had a heart attack. Carl had been admitted to the hospital three times for chest pain, and was placed in the cardiac intensive-care unit for observation in each case. But none of these episodes of chest pain was found to be a heart attack.

During this fourth hospitalization Carl underwent a cardiac catheterization. The test revealed that his heart was totally healthy. Carl had no heart disease! His chest pain proved later to be the result of excessive acid in his stomach, commonly called heartburn.

Some people will relate any pain in their chest to their heart. Carl assumed that he had had multiple heart attacks, because of the attention and monitoring that he received when he had had chest pain. But he was eventually discovered to have a healthy heart. Unfortunately, the reverse situation, ignoring chest pain, is more common and much more dangerous.

It is not always easy to tell where chest pain comes from. The common possibilities include: 1. ulcers or stomach irritation; 2. gallstones; 3. spasm of the esophagus (the food pipe connecting the throat to the stomach); 4. pneumonia and other lung conditions; and 5. irritation or injury to the muscles of the chest wall.

Each of these different conditions can result in pain that mimics a heart attack. It is difficult for experienced doctors to separate different types of chest pain, even after sophisticated testing. This is where clinical judgment plays a major role. It is better to *assume* that pain is from the heart, until proven otherwise.

Myth #3:
An attack of "angina" is the same thing as a heart attack.

Not all pain from the heart means that there is death of heart muscle. Angina is the pain that results when the heart muscle does not get enough blood (and oxygen) to do the work it is doing. This usually occurs during physical activity or emotional upset, each of which is a time when the heart works harder.

If there is a blockage in an artery of the heart (atherosclerosis), the supply of fuel might not be enough to meet the increased demand. This usually results in chest pain. But the heart muscle does not die, because it still receives some blood (even if the supply is less than it wants).

Stopping the exercise and/or taking heart medications usually suffice to end an episode of angina. Patients may experience daily episodes of angina, whereas heart attacks are much less common, and much more serious.

Myth #4:
A normal electrocardiogram ("cardiogram," EKG) means that a person is not having a heart attack.

This myth is a dangerous one.

Hank G., a forty-three-year-old insurance salesman, smoked two packs of cigarettes a day. His father died of a heart attack at the age of fifty-two. Hank had never been seriously ill. Yet one night he went to a local emergency room complaining of chest "tightness" lasting two hours, and mild nausea. An electrocardiogram was performed, and proved normal. Hank was reassured by the emergency room doctor that this was *not* a heart attack, and was sent home.

Hank told his wife, "Everything is okay. My cardiogram is normal."

He died one hour after arriving home.

Hank was having a heart attack, even though his electrocardiogram was normal. Although most people have classic changes on their EKG during an acute heart attack, many do not. These people will have heart attacks with normal or nearly normal EKG. And, like Hank, some are sent home inappropriately.

Some patients will have a normal EKG at the beginning of a heart attack, and will not demonstrate the characteristic abnormalities until several hours later. It is therefore wise to repeat the EKG before sending patients home: it may have changed while they were waiting in the emergency room. Other patients *never* demonstrate abnormalities on their EKG during a heart attack. Although this is very uncommon, these patients can die from a heart attack just as easily as those with the classic EKG findings.

A normal EKG should not have been completely reassuring to either Hank or his doctor in the emergency room. He should have been admitted to a cardiac-care unit for observation. His report of "cardiaclike" chest discomfort was serious enough to warrant hospitalization and careful monitoring in spite of the normal EKG. The EKG is not the beginning and end of diagnosis. It is not a perfect tool.

Myth #5:
If one has a "normal" stress test, one is not going to have a heart attack.

Robert K., a fifty-two-year-old man, had a stress test prior to joining a health club. He smoked one pack of cigarettes a day, but was otherwise in good health. His doctor recommended the test to be sure "it was all right to exercise." Robert passed the test with flying colors.

One month later he had a heart attack.

Robert had an atherosclerotic plaque in one of his coronary arteries just before his heart attack. It was present at the time of his stress test as well. But a stress test (also called an exercise test) will be normal in most people as long as the blockage is 50 percent or less.

In spite of its severity, a blockage of 50 percent will usually permit enough blood to reach the heart muscle to fuel all its activities. During a stress test, a patient walks on a treadmill machine that runs at faster and faster speeds, pushing the heart to work harder. If one of the arteries is more than 50 percent narrowed, the heart muscle eventually demands more fuel than the narrowed artery can now supply. This creates stress on the heart, which results in chest discomfort and changes in the electrocardiogram.

The result of a stress test will be normal (the heart reveals no stress during the exercise) as long as the heart gets enough fuel to do the extra work. If it is normal, we can assume that either the arteries are normal, or the blockages are minimal (less than 50 percent). But minimal plaque can abruptly occlude, leading to a heart attack. These minimal narrowings will not affect the result of a stress test, but they can still rupture, form blood clots, and result in heart attacks.

Most people who pass a stress test will not have heart attacks in the near future. A favorable test offers a statistical reassurance that things should be okay. But there are no absolute guarantees, especially among cigarette smokers. Smokers like Robert are more likely to develop clots in minimally diseased arteries, because the blood is more sticky.

Myth #6:
One heart attack is bad. But having a second or a third
will leave one as "a cripple."

The number of heart attacks is not as important as the total amount of heart muscle that has been damaged. Having a single large heart attack can be significantly worse than experiencing two small heart attacks. This is demonstrated by comparing the following two cases:

Mark T., a fifty-four-year-old man, experienced two heart attacks; the first occurred when he was forty-eight, involving the bottom wall of his heart. The total amount of damage was very small. Mark quit smoking, changed his diet, lost weight, and did everything right.

Despite this, six years later he had a second heart attack. Once again the damage occurred to a section of the bottom wall of his heart. Mark was very depressed. "I did everything I was told, so why did I have a second heart attack?"

Mark had the ejection fraction of his heart (left ventricle) measured, which was found to be 42 percent. Although the bottom wall of the left ventricle did not move, the other four walls were strong and healthy. Mark recovered without any symptoms and was ultimately able to resume all activities, taking only one medication for his heart. He is currently alive and well.

In contrast, Paul S., a sixty-three-year-old man, suffered a single massive heart attack involving the front wall of his heart. His ejection fraction was measured at 22 percent. Paul was greatly debilitated by this heart attack. He could not return to his job as a construction worker. He was tired and weak. He was left with a terrible prognosis.

Paul died less than three months after going home from the hospital.

Although Mark had suffered two heart attacks, both were tiny. The net amount of damage was very small, and his prognosis was excellent. He was not debilitated. In fact, after a recuperative period Mark was able to resume all of his usual activities. In contrast, Paul died after only one large heart attack.

Myth #7:
After a heart attack, one can't have sex.

This is a common fear, crossing the minds of most people recovering from heart attacks. Yet most people are afraid to ask their doctor about sex. There have been several celebrated examples of people (mainly men) dying during sexual encounters. A widespread perception exists that sex is dangerous for people who have heart disease. The sexual partners of people with heart disease are also afraid to resume sexual activity.

But sex is certainly *not* out of the question after a heart attack. The heart must first heal (from six to ten weeks) before any vigorous activity should be resumed. But afterward most people can handle the so-called stress of exercise and sex.

Sexual activity should be resumed gradually, and under a doctor's general guidelines. The amount of stress that sex places on the heart depends on many physical and psychological factors, and varies individually for each patient and his or her sexual partner.

Those with the largest amounts of heart-muscle damage may have difficulty with sexual performance. An extremely weak heart may not be able to meet the demands of the body during exercise. The patient may be too fatigued to engage in sex. Some men will be unable to obtain, or maintain, an erection if the cardiac output is too depressed.

Other patients develop anginal chest pain during sexual activity, because of blockages in the remaining arteries of their heart. Many will require medications to prevent these symptoms.

Sexual dysfunction can be caused or worsened by some cardiac medications. In this case stopping or changing the drugs might solve the problems. But this must be done under a doctor's direct supervision.

The psychological impact of having had a heart attack can be tremendous, playing a significant role in sexual difficulty thereafter. Counseling and reassurance make a big difference during the period of convalescence.

Fortunately, most people, after having had a heart attack, will not have trouble resuming a healthy sex life.

Myth #8:
It is bad to upset someone who has had a heart attack.
He or she might die.

This is also a common fear. But most people with heart disease are able to handle emotional stress without difficulty. It is reasonable to try to keep things calm, but this is not always possible. Sometimes trying to shelter a loved one can be more upsetting than allowing him or her to face some stress, particularly when trying to force people to "forget about work."

It is best to allow some patients to be involved with work from the hospital or home during the recovery period. This may prove to be less stressful than efforts to prevent it. Obviously it requires a case-by-case evaluation.

Stress is part of the real world. Patients with heart disease can't be hidden from stress forever. Luckily this is not a problem for most people who have had a heart attack. Eventually things return to normal with friends and family, and the usual disagreements and arguments occur anyway.

Myth #9:
A severely narrowed artery is definitely going to close off and cause a heart attack. An artery that is not critically narrowed is safe.

Brenda N., a sixty-five-year-old woman, was discovered to have a 90 percent narrowing of one of her three coronary arteries. She was told by her doctor that the artery "was hanging by a thread," and that a heart attack might be "around the corner." Although the patient felt well, she was advised to have the artery fixed by balloon angioplasty.

This is far from certain. Although one of the coronary arteries is 90 percent narrowed by atherosclerotic plaque, it is not just waiting to obstruct totally with a blood clot. Brenda may have had this 90 percent blockage for several years. The degree of narrowing does not predict the likelihood of blood-clot formation. A 50 percent plaque has the same potential as a 90 percent plaque to have a blood clot form on its surface, resulting in a heart attack.

Blood clots form under one of two conditions: 1. if the surface of the plaque breaks or ruptures, making it unstable; or 2. if the entire clotting system becomes excessively active. These events do not depend on the degree of narrowing of the atherosclerosis.

Brenda, whose chest pain was predictable and under control (stable angina), is likely to remain stable. She has little to gain prognostically by having her artery "fixed," even though it is 90 percent narrowed. On the other hand, a patient whose chest pain occurs with less and less exertion (unstable angina) is more likely to have the beginning of clot formation. Even if the coronary artery is less significantly narrowed, this patient would have more to gain by undergoing a repair of the artery.

Clot-Busting Drugs

The formation of a blood clot is ultimately responsible for occluding an artery and starting a heart attack. Consequently, drugs capable of dissolving clots have been explored as a means to open up an occluded artery and restore blood flow to the heart muscle. These new drugs, the clot-busting drugs, have been proven very successful. They have been demonstrated to save heart muscle and lives.

Bigger heart attacks are associated with a worsened likelihood of survival. It would be ideal if we could prevent heart attacks in the first place. But this is not always possible. Therefore, much of our effort has been directed at reducing the size of heart attacks *once they begin*.

Many drugs and strategies have been explored during the

past two decades to accomplish this goal, but most had very disappointing results. Only one approach has been found to be successful—the use of the clot-busting drugs, called thrombolytic agents.

When a coronary artery becomes abruptly occluded by a blood clot, a section of heart muscle becomes deprived of all blood flow. The cells of that section of muscle begin to die. But they don't die right away. They take several hours to die. During these critical hours, restoring blood flow can rescue these dying muscle cells.

Restoring blood flow within twenty minutes of an occlusion is likely to prevent completely the death of heart muscle, although it is rare for anyone to be within medical reach this early. Opening the artery within one hour will limit the amount of injury to approximately 50 percent of the muscle at risk.

As time goes by more and more heart cells die. The earlier a patient gets to the hospital, the greater the amount of the heart is still alive and available to be saved. It takes from three to six hours for a heart attack to be completed. After this time almost all the jeopardized heart muscle has died.

Currently there are two drugs approved by the Food and Drug Administration that are available to dissolve clots during heart attacks. They are called streptokinase and tissue plasminogen activator (TPA). These drugs have no effect on the underlying atherosclerotic plaque. The best that they can accomplish is to eliminate all the clot, leaving the artery with its underlying narrowing.

The artery might be 99 percent obstructed by plaque, but by eliminating the clot some blood flow will be restored down the artery. Even this very limited blood flow will be enough to rescue some of the dying heart muscle.

Myth #10:
The new clot-busting drugs will save the lives of everybody having a heart attack.

There is little doubt that these new drugs can and do save lives. But, like all medical tools, they are not perfect. Some people will die despite therapy with a clot-busting medication. Two European scientific studies examined these questions.

An Italian study, called GISSI[2] (Gruppo Italiano Per Lo Studio Della Streptochinasi Nell'Infarto Miocardico), involved more than 11,000 men and women having heart attacks. The already noted study ISIS[3] (International Study of Infarct Survival), conducted in northern Europe, involved more than 17,000 patients. These two studies overshadow in size almost all other clinical investigations of heart disease, making them extremely valuable. The results are striking.

The studies were very similar. In both, patients were randomly assigned to either streptokinase therapy (administered through an intravenous line) or an inactive placebo. The patients were otherwise treated equally, and were given standard therapy for heart attacks. The object was to determine whether administration of streptokinase reduced the number of patients dying during the period of hospitalization.

Receiving streptokinase, especially early in the course of a heart attack, saved lives in both studies. The following table demonstrates the results of giving patients streptokinase within three hours of the onset of the heart attack (which is assumed to coincide with the beginning of chest pain):

RECEIVING DRUG WITHIN 3 HOURS:
HOSPITAL DEATH RATE

	PLACEBO	STREPTOKINASE
GISSI	12.0%	9.2%
ISIS	12.2%	8.1%

Receiving streptokinase within the first hour of chest pain produced the most dramatic results, as demonstrated in the following table. Unfortunately, most patients (approximately 95 percent) did not get to the hospital until *after* one hour of chest pain.

RECEIVING DRUG WITHIN 1 HOUR:
HOSPITAL DEATH RATE

	PLACEBO	STREPTOKINASE
GISSI	15.4%	8.2%
ISIS	13.4%	8.1%

In both studies the patients receiving streptokinase had significantly fewer deaths than the patients receiving the placebo. The death rate among the people given the placebo ranged from 12 percent to 15 percent. This is approximately the same average death rate for people experiencing heart attack in the United States. The use of streptokinase reduced this mortality down to 8 or 9 percent.

In the ISIS study some patients were given a combination of streptokinase and aspirin (one adult tablet a day) when they got to the emergency room. This combination proved to be significantly better than giving streptokinase alone, further reducing the death rate to 6.5 percent!

The other FDA-approved thrombolytic drug, TPA, may prove to be as (or even more) effective in saving lives. However, the information is not yet available to assess the effect of TPA on heart attack survival. It is a newer drug, and has not been as extensively tested as streptokinase. We expect the results of some important comparative studies in the very near future.

In summary, approximately 12 percent of all heart attack victims will die in the hospital while receiving otherwise standard medical care. With the use of thrombolytic drugs, this death rate is reduced to roughly 9 percent (although the additional use of aspirin may further drop mortality down to 6 percent). Thus, from 3 percent, up to 6 percent, of patients will have their lives saved by treatment with clot-busting drugs if therapy is begun within three hours of the heart attack.

Only half of all people having heart attacks come to a hospital within three or four hours of the beginning of chest pain. The other half (more than 350,000 people a year) reach the hospital too late to receive these clot-busting drugs. Further, thrombolytic therapy works best when administered within one hour of chest pain; yet only 5 percent of all patients reach the hospital this early. More people could receive this therapy, and more lives could be saved, it those having heart attacks received medical attention more quickly.

The majority of patients will not derive any survival benefit from treatment with the drug, even if they reach the hospital within three hours. But no one patient can tell in advance whether he or she will be one of the lucky 3 percent to have their lives saved. As a result, we recommend the use of thrombolytic therapy to most eligible patients experiencing acute heart attacks.

Some patients are at greater risk of complications with clot-busting therapy than others. In general we avoid the use of these drugs in people who: 1. are older than seventy-five years of age; 2. have had recent surgery; 3. have active bleeding problems (like a bleeding ulcer); and 4. have had recent strokes (these drugs can cause bleeding in the brain). In many of these patients the risks of therapy outweigh the potential benefits, and thus we will not use the drugs.

Even in otherwise healthy people the biggest risk from receiving clot-busting drugs is serious and potentially life-threatening bleeding. These drugs work because they dissolve clots within the arteries of the heart. But they also dissolve clots in other parts of the body. This can produce bleeding anywhere from the site of an intravenous line to a previously healed ulcer in the stomach. A blood transfusion was required in more than 5 out of every 1,000 people treated in the European studies. The most devastating complication is bleeding into the brain (which occurs in at least 2 out of every 1,000 patients treated with streptokinase), resulting in a stroke or death. TPA may have an even higher incidence of producing cerebral bleeding.

But even with these complications, the total number of deaths will be reduced among patients who are treated with thrombolytic therapy. Although there is clearly a risk involved when giving these drugs, for the average patient there is an even greater risk in *not* giving them.

There are no guarantees. We can't save the life of everyone having a heart attack, even if the person goes quickly to the hospital (9 percent of patients will die despite clot-busting therapy). The use of thrombolytic drugs will improve the statistical chance of survival for any given patient.

In the United States there are 750,000 people hospitalized each year with heart attacks. We predict that roughly 90,000 will die during the initial hospitalization. The widespread use of thrombolytic therapy could potentially save up to 22,000 lives every year. But this would require that all patients reach the hospital within three hours of having chest pain.

Although we have spent a great deal of time and money, and done much research to find ways to reduce the mortality of the people who reach the hospital (90,000 deaths each year), this is only the tip of the iceberg. Most cardiac deaths occur before the victim reaches the hospital (300,000 deaths each year). Tragically, many of these deaths might have been prevented had the patient quickly reached medical attention. Some lives could even be saved after an episode of sudden death.

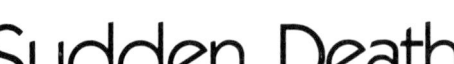

CHAPTER SIX

Sudden Death

Each year in the United States 300,000 people die suddenly from heart disease. These people die without warning, and without time to do anything. People often assume, or merely hope, that if they develop heart disease they will have time to do something about it. But many will not have this luxury.

Myth #1:
"If I am going to get heart problems, I'll have a warning first. I'll have time to do something."

This is not always true! More than 25 percent of heart patients first learn that they have a problem by dying suddenly.

Eric L., a forty-two-year-old man, smoked two packs of cigarettes a day. "I know I should quit," he told his doctor at his last checkup. "I'll do it at the end of the year, when things at work slow down." Although he was not particularly active, he felt well.

Two weeks after his checkup, he collapsed while leaving work. When the paramedics arrived he was dead, and could not be resuscitated. The autopsy revealed that he had suffered an acute heart attack. He never knew there was a problem.

His wife was stunned. "He was never sick. How could this happen?"

Eric had smoked cigarettes, putting him at a much higher than average risk for experiencing a premature heart attack. He never had a chance to quit smoking or to attempt other life-style modifications. A great many people who have heart attacks, and who experience sudden death, are caught completely by surprise. They thought of themselves as healthy before the acute event.

Myth #2:
Once your heart stops, you're dead. It's too late
to do anything.

Sudden death is not necessarily a permanent condition. Sometimes after the heart stops beating (called a cardiac arrest) it can be started again. If the heart is restarted quickly (within minutes of the cardiac arrest), the victim's life can be saved. Unfortunately, this usually requires sophisticated medical equipment and medications.

If the heart stands still too long, it will be too late to save the patient. The lack of blood flow throughout the rest of the body will result in the death of the brain and other vital organs.

Fortunately, there is a way to buy time until the sophisticated help arrives. Cardio-pulmonary resuscitation (CPR) is a technique that can keep blood and oxygen flowing in a person's body while his or her heart is not working. CPR is performed by pumping on the victim's chest (literally squeezing the blood through the heart) and breathing into the victim's mouth, thus delivering oxygen into the lungs. Anyone can take a class and learn how to perform CPR.

Myth #3:
CPR will bring someone back to life after he or she has experienced cardiac arrest.

This is not true. CPR does not bring people back to life. The name itself, cardio-pulmonary *resuscitation,* is misleading: there is no resuscitation involved. The technique is intended to keep blood flowing until medical help arrives. If this help does not arrive, the patient will die. CPR will not, by itself, start the heart beating again, nor bring someone back to life after cardiac arrest.

Many people do not realize this, and assume that it is CPR that resuscitates a patient. Of course, without CPR there would not be a chance for rescue. Most people need this support, because sophisticated medical help usually takes more than several minutes to arrive. CPR is therefore vital.

Even with effective CPR, and even with immediate medical attention, not everyone can have his or her heart started again after cardiac arrest. Success depends mainly on why it has stopped beating in the first place.

Myth #4:
Sudden cardiac death is the same event for all patients.

Most people assume that when the heart stops, it is for the same reason in different people. Sudden death is lumped together as a single problem, or disease.

But it does not occur for only one reason. There are, instead, two basic mechanisms or categories of sudden death: 1. mechanical failure; and 2. electrical failure. The heart can stop because of a heart attack, a bad reaction to drugs, or from a profound mineral imbalance in the blood. But regardless of the *underlying* cause, the ultimate mechanism is either electrical or mechanical.

We have a good chance of rescuing a heart that has stopped beating because of an electrical problem, and virtually no chance if it has stopped for mechanical reasons. But even if the heart has stopped because of a treatable, electrical problem, the patient may not survive if CPR is ineffective or initiated too late.

If a person collapses in the street (or in the hospital) and is found without a pulse, it is not possible to tell if the problem is mechanical or electrical. If it is mechanical, the person almost certainly cannot be saved. But because we do not know which is the case, we initiate CPR, hoping for the best. Time is critical. Delaying CPR can make the difference between success and failure.

Therefore, if a patient experiences sudden death we recommend CPR in all cases, and make all efforts to save the person's life. Only later, if the person survives (or by autopsy if he or she dies), can we try to figure out what happened.

Most of the mechanical problems are related to acute heart attacks. In contrast, a large number of the electrical problems are unrelated. Some people with chronic, otherwise "stable" heart disease will experience electrical instability, without suffering an acute heart attack. These differences will now be explained, starting with the mechanical failure of the heart.

Mechanical Failure

Mechanical failure is exactly what the name implies. It occurs when the heart muscle physically fails to pump blood to the rest of the body.

Ken C., a sixty-three-year-old man, suffered from a huge heart attack. His ejection fraction was found to be 15 percent on his second day in the hospital. Over the next few days, he felt weaker and weaker, and his blood pressure began to drop. His kidneys began to fail, and he became progressively more confused.

Ken died in the hospital three days after his heart attack. Efforts to resuscitate him were unsuccessful.

This form of mechanical heart failure is directly related to the amount of muscle damaged during a heart attack. If 30 percent to 40 percent of the heart muscle has been destroyed, the patient will usually die. The cardiac output (the amount of blood pumped by the heart) is diminished because of the large loss of heart muscle. The rest of the body fails to receive enough blood to function normally, resulting in profound weakness, and ultimately death. The patient can't be resuscitated, because the death of muscle is irreversible, and the heart has given in.

The muscle of the heart can be damaged by things other than heart attacks. High blood pressure puts stress on the heart muscle and, over many years, can lead to failure of the heart. Alcohol, certain drugs, and some viral illness can also damage heart muscle, resulting in mechanical failure in the most severe cases.

A different form of mechanical failure, "cardiac rupture," is not directly related to the amount of muscle that has died during a heart attack. The literal rupture of a wall of the heart is a very sudden, catastrophic, and tragic complication. It can complicate even a small heart attack, because it does not require a great deal of muscle injury.

This form of mechanical failure frequently comes as a complete surprise. Before the rupture, the heart is working well without signs of difficulty. Suddenly, without warning, one of the walls of the heart abruptly tears open resulting in instantaneous death.

Ted G., a forty-nine-year-old man, had a medium-sized heart attack, involving the front wall of his heart. His ejection fraction afterward was 38 percent. He had an uneventful hospital course and was discharged on the eighth day after admission. The next day, at home, he died suddenly. He had been feeling well just before his death, and had not complained to his family of anything that day. An autopsy revealed that the front wall of his heart had torn open, resulting in his sudden death.

Cardiac rupture is most likely to occur during a three-week "vulnerable period" immediately following a heart attack. Within a few days the body begins to clear away the recently killed muscle from the heart. This clearing process weakens the wall of the heart (large sections of dead muscle are removed), making it vulnerable to rupture.

During the next few weeks the wall regains strength, as the body replaces the dead muscle with scar tissue (forming a patch in the heart). Scar tissue is very strong, and very difficult to tear open and rupture.

During the period of waiting for the formation of scar tissue, the wall of the heart is at risk for rupture. Physical stress is dangerous during this period of healing, which is why we recommend that activity be limited during the first few weeks after a heart attack. Even if a patient feels well, the wall of the heart needs to heal without stress, and the patient should remain somewhat sedentary for several weeks. Once the wall strengthens, more activity is allowed.

Fortunately, this disastrous complication of rupture occurs in only 1 percent to 2 percent of people who have had heart attacks. It is almost always fatal, although there are occasional reports of a person's surviving cardiac rupture because of immediate surgery. But this is quite rare. Most patients would not survive even if they were immediately rushed into the operating room.

Electrical Failure

The heart is more likely to be saved if cardiac arrest is caused by an electrical malfunction. The heart has a sophisticated electrical system vital to its function. It requires an electrical signal for the muscle to work and beat.

This electrical system is necessary for life. The heart must repeatedly receive electrical signals to work. And the muscle must further receive this signal in an organized way. If the electric signal were to reach different parts of the heart muscle at different times, the walls would contract without synchrony, and the heart would fail to pump blood forward effectively (which depends on the walls squeezing together).

If the electrical system becomes interrupted or disorganized, the result can be cardiac arrest and death. But, unlike most of the mechanical problems, these electrical problems can usually be successfully treated.

The majority of all sudden cardiac deaths results from the disorganization of the electrical system of the heart, which is somewhat akin to a short circuit. "Electrical" deaths can be provoked by many types of stress, such as profound changes in the mineral content of the blood, by bad reactions to certain medications, and by the presence of scar tissue in the heart muscle.

Heart attacks can also be responsible for cases of electrical death. The interruption of blood flow to a section of heart muscle causes both the death of that muscle and instability of the electrical system.

The dying cells of the heart muscle break apart, releasing dangerous chemicals and minerals capable of disrupting the normal, orderly spread of electricity. This can result in a totally chaotic rhythm called "ventricular fibrillation."

Ventricular fibrillation is lethal. It is equivalent to a complete short circuit of the electrical system of the heart, in which there is the random, disorganized spread of electricity. The muscle stops beating, resulting in sudden death.

Ventricular fibrillation can be converted back to normal by delivering an electrical shock to the heart, which, amazingly, "resets" the electrical system, returning things to normal. Because we can't deliver a shock directly to the heart, we instead send the electric impulse across the chest wall, which then travels inward to the heart muscle.

This is done with a special machine called a defibrillator, which uses round metal paddles charged with an electric current (usually 300 watt-seconds of current). The paddles are placed on the chest wall, then triggered to release their electric discharge. And, just like in the movies, the patient's body jumps up. This happens because the electric impulse spreads throughout the rest of the body, stimulating the muscles of the arms and legs to contract abruptly.

The electric shock from the defibrillator spreads throughout the heart muscle and resets the electrical system, usually back to normal. Sometimes a second, or even a third, shock is required to return order to the electrical system. The amount of electric current delivered usually will not damage the heart, and a person can safely undergo multiple shocks if necessary.

If the heart stops for mechanical reasons, it is *not* likely to respond to an electric shock, because the problem is not electrical. However, if there is a primary electrical problem, such as ventricular fibrillation during a heart attack, the results can be dramatic.

Jane G., a sixty-two-year-old woman, knew something was wrong when she abruptly developed "crushing" chest pain while reading a book at home. She began to sweat and feel light-headed. She called the paramedics to come to her house.

Soon after the ambulance arrived, Jane suffered from cardiac arrest, because she developed ventricular fibrillation. She was promptly administered a shock of electricity (300 watt-seconds) across her chest from the electric defibrillator, and her heart's rhythm returned to normal.

The paramedics placed an intravenous line into Jane's arm and injected lidocaine (a drug that helps to prevent future episodes of ventricular fibrillation).

Jane was very lucky. If she had not called the paramedics she would certainly have died, because ventricular fibrillation requires an electrical shock to convert the heart's rhythm back to normal. Furthermore, Jane was treated within seconds of her cardiac arrest, improving the odds of successful therapy.

Each year tens of thousands of people die from ventricular fibrillation, before help arrives. Tragically, many could be saved by rapid electrical defibrillation.

In Seattle, Washington, an interesting experiment was performed to examine the importance of rapid defibrillation.[1] It was observed that fire fighters were often the first to arrive on the scene of a cardiac arrest, even before the paramedics.

Fire fighters were trained in CPR, but were not trained to use the electric defibrillator (which was thus not available until the paramedics arrive).

However, an easy-to-use, automatic defibrillator was issued to one-half of the city's fire fighters. It contained a computer chip that was programmed to automatically deliver an electric shock to the patient if it detected ventricular fibrillation. The fireman was responsible only for attaching the device to the victim.

The automatic defibrillator provided the opportunity to give a patient an electric shock (if needed) prior to the arrival of the paramedics. The aim of the study was to determine if this approach would save lives.

During 1987, in Seattle, there were 228 episodes of sudden death in which fire fighters arrived first and administered traditional CPR until the arrival of the paramedics. Among these patients, 19 percent survived.

In contrast, 30 percent of 276 patients survived if the fire fighters, who arrived first, used the automatic defibrillator. A greater number of these patients survived because of the early opportunity for electric defibrillation.

Of note, the study further demonstrated the importance of bystander CPR. The likelihood of survival was four times greater if CPR was initiated immediately, when compared to the times when it was delayed (such as when the collapse was not witnessed).

When CPR was initiated within four minutes, and the defibrillator was available within eight minutes, the survival rate was greater than 40 percent! In contrast, late CPR (after eight minutes) followed by late defibrillation (after sixteen minutes) resulted in approximately 0 percent survival. Even with early CPR, if defibrillator use was delayed beyond eight minutes, the prognosis became progressively more dismal.

This opens up the question of whether the wider availability of the automatic defibrillator to the public could save even more lives. This is not easy to answer. Certainly many of the 300,000 sudden deaths each year could be avoided by both bystander CPR and rapid defibrillation.

A middle-aged man collapsed in a restaurant. Two patrons began CPR immediately, while others called for an ambulance. The paramedics arrived fifteen minutes later and found the heart in ventricular fibrillation. Despite several electric shocks administered with the defibrillator, they failed to convert the man's rhythm back to normal.

Although he received speedy CPR, there was a significant delay in the arrival of the paramedics. If an automatic defibrillator had been available, perhaps in the restaurant, his life might have been saved.

This is a complex issue with many medical, social, and legal ramifications. The widespread availability of automatic defibrillators would clearly save some lives. But the machines are expensive, and there would be problems related to machine malfunction. Because computer circuits are not perfect, eventually there would be reports of a person's receiving an unnecessary electric shock, for example, after a mere fainting spell. Legislation would be needed to protect the untrained public who might use this machine.

On a more limited scale, family members of high-risk patients could be trained to use these devices. This could save the lives of some people in their homes. But even this approach is expensive.

For the present time, the public should be as widely trained as possible in CPR. This is especially recommended for family members of those with serious heart disease. CPR, when performed according to standard training, is vital to a successful resuscitation.

Unfortunately, the fear of contracting AIDS has contributed to the reluctance of the public to perform mouth-to-mouth breathing (an essential part of CPR) on strangers. Even so, masks are available that can protect a person from direct mouth-to-mouth contact, yet still permit effective respiratory resuscitation. One breathes into the mask, which is placed on the victim's mouth. These masks are not very expensive, and should be made more widely available.

Over 25 percent of people admitted to the hospital with heart attacks will experience ventricular fibrillation and sudden death. However, we can prevent this electrical instability before it occurs in people admitted with acute heart attacks.

Certain drugs are available, like the drug lidocaine, which prevent ventricular fibrillation during the acute heart attack. These drugs, technically called "anti-arrhythmic" drugs, stabilize the electric system of the heart. They can usually prevent ventricular fibrillation, but are not effective at converting an episode back to normal if it occurs. These patients still require the addition of an electric shock.

Ventricular fibrillation would complicate 30 percent of all heart attacks, but the routine use of lidocaine has prevented the majority of these episodes before they occur. Some patients will experience ventricular fibrillation despite this protective therapy, and require emergent electrical defibrillation in the hospital. This is why every patient in a cardiac-care unit is on a monitor, and has an electric defibrillator at his or her bedside.

The electrical instability of the heart is greatest during the first forty-eight hours after the onset of a heart attack. Things quiet down afterward. Hence, the protective drugs are usually stopped after the second hospital day.

Ventricular fibrillation (and sudden death) can occur in people besides those having a heart attack. There are other reasons for the degeneration of the cardiac rhythm, such as the presence of scar tissue in the heart.

As dead muscle heals from an earlier heart attack, scar tissue is created. Over the years, this scar tissue disrupts the flow of electricity around it. It can, without warning, cause a sudden and fatal change of heart rhythm. Whereas ventricular fibrillation during an acute heart attack is the result of the chemicals released during the first forty-eight hours, scar tissue is a chronic and much less predictable problem.

Burt D., a fifty-nine-year-old man who had a large heart attack involving the front wall, was found to have an ejection fraction of 24 percent. He eventually returned to work and resumed most of his usual activities, although he felt slower.

Burt collapsed three years later while at work. His secretary, finding no pulse, began CPR. The paramedics arrived within twelve minutes and, finding Burt in ventricular fibrillation, immediately used the paddles to administer an electric shock across his chest. The first shock failed to change his rhythm, but a second shock proved successful. They then administered a dose of lidocaine.

Burt became conscious and was brought to the hospital. His electrocardiogram was without new changes, and his blood tests were all normal.

Burt suffered from ventricular fibrillation (and nearly died), but did *not* have another heart attack, and was *not* involved in physical activity at the time of his cardiac arrest. Although Burt was at work, he was otherwise comfortable and relaxed.

Ventricular fibrillation can occur many years after a heart

attack. Scar tissue (remaining from the heart attack) creates electrical instability in the surrounding muscle. These patients commonly have extra beats of electricity, created by the scar tissue, called ventricular premature contractions (VPCs).

The VPCs are generated in addition to the electricity coming from the heart's natural pacemaker (called the sinus node). They are described by patients as "extra" beats, and are usually harmless. However, if several of these extra beats are rapidly generated in a row, they can cause an electrical short circuit, resulting in ventricular fibrillation.

Myth #5:
Extra beats are bad for everybody, and should always be treated.

Multiple VPCs are more dangerous in people with weakened hearts because they are more vulnerable to electrical disruption. Those with healthy and strong hearts rarely develop ventricular fibrillation, and the VPCs are less threatening and do not require therapy.

Carol B., a thirty-two-year-old woman who complained of palpitations, was discovered to have multiple VPCs, with many of them occurring in rapid sequence (called ventricular tachycardia). She underwent a battery of medical tests; her heart muscle was strong and healthy, and she had a normal exercise test.

Carol's physician was convinced that she was at a great risk for sudden death and wanted her to undergo a more sophisticated, "invasive" cardiac evaluation. Carol requested a second opinion, and was told that she had nothing to worry about.

She went home without submitting to the invasive tests and without taking any medications. It took her months to realize that she was not dying every time she felt a palpitation. The warnings from her first doctor had haunted her.

In a young patient without underlying heart disease, extra beats are harmless, although many physicians do not realize this. Carol was not at an increased risk from her VPCs, and did not require further testing or medications. On the other hand, patients with underlying coronary artery disease, with previous heart attacks, and with weakened heart muscles are at a significantly greater risk from VPCs. These people are much more susceptible to ventricular fibrillation and sudden death. In this population, VPCs are the harbinger of serious problems.

Lenny D., a fifty-eight-year-old man, had a large heart attack. His ejection fraction was moderately depressed below normal (34 percent), and he was discovered to have frequent VPCs, with occasional "runs" of consecutive VPCs (ventricular tachycardia).

In contrast to Carol, Lenny is at high risk for sudden death because of the presence of VPCs (he has up to a 20 percent chance of dying suddenly every year). Surprisingly, treating the VPCs with drugs does not prevent sudden death. These people still experience sudden death despite the anti-arrhythmic drug therapy.

The drugs used to suppress extra beats work by altering the heart's electrical system, but they often do so in unpredictable ways. For example, they can cause electrical instability, and ventricular fibrillation, instead of suppressing them, which is known as a "pro-arrhythmic" effect.

It is ironic that drugs used to treat a problem can, in fact, make the problem more serious and more likely to occur. Up to 60 percent of people who are resuscitated from out-of-hospital sudden death are found to be taking an anti-arrhythmic drug at the time of their cardiac arrest. The sudden death had occurred either because of or despite their medication. Every drug, clinically used, has the potential both to help and cause harm, and they should be used with caution.

Many doctors will prescribe an anti-arrhythmic drug (procainamide the most common one) for a heart attack patient if the presence of extra beats is detected. But this approach is outdated, and potentially dangerous. There is no evidence that using drugs will prevent sudden death, and such drugs can be dangerous. We do not recommend anti-arrhythmic drug therapy for most people who have had heart attacks, even if they have extra beats. However, some people do require therapy with anti-arrhythmic drugs.

People who have been resuscitated from a sudden death experience have up to a 40 percent rate of recurrent sudden death within two years of the initial episode. Physicians recommend that these high-risk people undergo an in-depth, and very specialized, evaluation of their heart's electrical system. The test is called "electrical program stimulation" (EPS).

In a laboratory, the heart is subjected to a predefined program of electrical stimulations. An electrical wire, under X-ray guidance, is inserted into the right-side chamber of the heart (through an intravenous line, following the return of blood back to the heart). Electric impulses are then transmitted through this wire to the heart muscle, mimicking the VPCs. These impulses are not felt by the patient. There is no pain. The electricity is delivered to the heart at an increasingly rapid rate, creating electrical stress, in an effort to duplicate the sudden-death experience by provoking a short circuit.

The test usually succeeds in inducing ventricular fibrillation and sudden death, which is immediately converted back to normal with an electric shock. The test is safe and effective. In nearly every case recorded to date in an EPS lab, the electricity has been returned to normal. The test is, nonetheless, frightening. But it is much more psychologically difficult to withstand than it is physically dangerous.

Once ventricular fibrillation has been induced by the EPS test, and reversed, an anti-arrhythmic drug is administered. The test is then repeated (after a large dose of the drug has been given). The drug is a success if it prevents the stimulation from, once again, inducing ventricular fibrillation. If the drug succeeds in the test, it is very likely to prevent sudden death outside of the hospital.

Burt D., the fifty-nine-year-old man who was saved from his sudden-death experience at work because of rapid and effective CPR, was urged to undergo EPS to define the problem, and so that the correct drug could be selected to treat him.

The study provoked ventricular fibrillation after relatively minimal electrical stimulation, causing him to experience sudden death in the laboratory. Burt became unconscious within seconds of his heart's stopping, and was immediately administered a 300-joule shock of electricity, which converted his rhythm back to normal. Although he felt no pain (he was unconscious at the time of the electric shock to his chest wall), Burt was very upset by the experience. He remembered "falling out," and was scared to let it happen again.

Burt was convinced by his doctors that he needed this study (he had already been lucky to survive sudden death outside the hospital, and was at grave risk for it to occur again). He was first treated with lidocaine, which was unable to prevent the electric stimulation from inducing ventricular fibrillation. He was then tested with several other drugs on different days (as one must wait for each drug to clear the system before testing the next one).

The fourth drug tested proved to be successful and the heart remained in normal rhythm even after the maximum electrical stimulation. Understandably, Burt was upset by these studies, but has since done well on his anti-arrhythmic medications. He continues to live a productive life.

Without the EPS test one can't be certain that any one drug will succeed in preventing arrhythmia in any one given patient. We can make an educated guess as to whether a chosen drug is effective. We can count the number of VPCs (extra beats) before giving a drug, then see if the number is greatly diminished after an adequate dose of the drug is given (this approach is considered non-invasive, whereas EPS is considered invasive). However, this non-invasive approach is not as reliable as the EPS method, which is the best way to assess the efficacy of a potential drug in a sudden-death survivor.

Individual drugs usually have only a 20 percent chance of successfully preventing recurrent sudden death for any given patient. Therefore, it is statistically likely that the first drug will fail the EPS test. In fact, many drugs must frequently be tested until the right one comes along. The need for multiple drug testing often makes the test extremely frustrating.

Sometimes all drugs fail in the test. If this is the case, then the patient is at risk for recurrent sudden death, and there is nothing we can do to prevent the arrhythmia. But we have a last resort. We can surgically insert a device, called an "implantable defibrillator," into these patients. This is a sophisticated instrument that continuously monitors the electrical rhythm of the heart. If it detects ventricular fibrillation, it automatically delivers a strong electrical discharge directly to the heart muscle. To do this, metal paddles are surgically implanted on the surface of the heart, with a power pack and computer microprocessor placed in the belly.

This device will deliver an electric shock to defibrillate these high-risk people after they develop recurrent fibrillation. It does not prevent the sudden death. It treats it. The devices have been proven to be quite successful and have saved many lives. But for those who can be managed with successful drug therapy, this more radical form of treatment is not required.

In some cases the location of the scar tissue in the heart muscle which is responsible for the electrical instability can be identified in the operating room. In select cases this abnormal section of the heart wall can be surgically removed. Although this type of surgery is very risky, it has the potential to cure a patient of their sudden death syndrome.

CHAPTER SEVEN

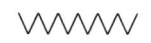

Palpitations and Pacemakers

We are usually unaware of the beating of our own heart. Except during heavy work or exercise, when we are accustomed to feeling a pounding in our chest, this sensation is a troubling reminder of our own mortality.

Many people experience palpitations, a symptom that is misunderstood. There are many myths concerning the rate at which the heart should beat, arrhythmias (which are alterations in the heart rate), and pacemakers. All these problems all relate to the heart rate.

Myth #1:
There is a "normal" heart rate.

Normal has been defined as any heart rate taken while a person is at rest that is between 60 and 100 beats per minute. A heart rate slower than 60 beats per minute is called bradycardia ("brady" means slow), while that which is faster than 100 beats per minute is called tachycardia ("tachy" means fast).

Some people have these faster or slower rates and are still very healthy. Although most people fall within the normal range, it is not an absolute requirement. As a general rule, if a person is unaware of his or her own heartbeat, then regardless of the rate, it is probably normal for him or her.

Alex F., a thirty-eight-year-old investment banker who exercised routinely at a health club, was troubled when his doctor told him that his heart rate was 52 beats per minute. Although Alex felt healthy, he was worried that his heartbeat was too slow and wondered if his heart might stop.

It is common for athletes like Alex to have a slower-than-average pulse rate, which is a healthy response. Although the heart is beating more slowly, it is actually beating more efficiently. In contrast:

Barry G., a fifty-four-year-old overweight office worker who rarely exercised, was found to have a heart rate of 102 beats per minute. He was unaware of his fast pulse until his most recent medical checkup.

Barry is in poor condition, and is "out of shape." Because his heart beats somewhat inefficiently, his heart rate is faster than normal, but it is not causing him to experience any symptoms. Although this tachycardia reflects his poor overall physical conditioning, it is not itself dangerous.

However, a heart rate of 102 beats per minute can be a problem for some patients:

Richard H., a sixty-two-year-old man with hardening of the arteries, had a pulse, while at rest, of 102 beats per minute.

His activity was greatly limited because he developed chest pain whenever his heart rate exceeded 110 beats per minute. When Richard was placed on medications that slowed his pulse, he found he could be more active.

Richard, because of his heart condition, can't tolerate the same heart rate that an otherwise healthy person can tolerate. More extreme variations in either direction will usually be poorly tolerated by everybody and can lead to severe symptoms, including chest pain, dizziness, fainting, and even sudden death. In these cases the fast or slow heart rate is no longer considered normal.

Maximum Heart Rate

Although normal varies from person to person, there appears to be a physiologic maximum rate that the heart can achieve. For children and adolescents this rate is approximately 200 beats per minute. Regardless of the level of activity, the human heart generally can't beat faster than this limit.

With increasing age, the heart slows down, and the maximum rate becomes lower and lower, which is estimated by the following formula:

$$\text{Maximum Heart Rate} = 200 \text{ minus } \tfrac{1}{2} \text{ Age}$$

For example, a fifty-year-old man, during exercise, can be expected to achieve a maximum heart rate of 175 beats per minute. (One-half of his age equals 25; 25 is then subtracted from 200, which equals 175). This is not an ironclad rule, but is rather a guideline used to predict the response of a healthy heart.

Most people, in day-to-day life, never reach their maximum heart rate. Even during heavy activity, most will approach only 70 percent to 80 percent of their maximum rate.

During exercise, when the heart rate becomes faster than 100 beats per minute, it is officially called a tachycardia, but is a normal physiologic response. Rates as high as 120 beats per minute to 150 beats per minute are common during heavy work, and are appropriate for the needs of the body.

On the other hand, a rate of 150 beats per minute should not occur in a person who is otherwise at rest. Yet, in some people, it does. These tachycardias occur because electric impulses in the heart are inappropriately generated. During such episodes, patients frequently complain of palpitations.

Myth #2:
There is a disease called "palpitations," which is very dangerous to have.

This is a common myth.

A palpitation is simply the awareness of the heart's beating—either more quickly or more intensely than normal. A doctor can't determine if a patient has palpitations, because it is a *symptom* (like a headache or an itch) that is experienced by the patient. A doctor can, however, determine *why* a patient experiences palpitations.

The sensation of pounding in the chest can be the result of a rapid heartbeat (tachycardia), or an irregular heart rate. In these cases, the electrical system of the heart needs to be evaluated. But in other patients palpitations are experienced during times that the heart is beating at a normal and steady rate. It is not understood why these patients have their symptoms when everything else checks out as normal. In these cases, reassurance is the only therapy.

Palpitations usually occur in self-limiting episodes, lasting from several seconds to hours. Most patients find that their episodes terminate before they are seen by a doctor, making it difficult to diagnose the underlying cause. A normal EKG after the fact is not very helpful.

The Twenty-four-Hour Monitor

Because it was recognized that most symptoms are experienced at home, a monitoring device was developed to be used outside of the doctor's office. The twenty-four-hour cardiac monitor (also called a Holter monitor) is a small electrocardiogram machine that runs for a complete day.

Electrodes are attached to the chest wall, and are connected to a small box that is worn over the shoulder, like a small tape recorder. The EKG is monitored continuously and stored on a magnetic tape. When the patient experiences a palpitation, he or she pushes a button on the side of the machine marking the moment.

After the machine is removed, the tape is reviewed by a doctor (with the help of a computer), and the heart rate can be examined for the entire twenty-four hours of the study. Special attention is given to the times the event marker was pushed.

When evaluating a patient who complains of palpitations, it is important to discover if there is an underlying cause. If there is no underlying heart problem, the patient can be reassured. If, on the other hand, a specific electrical disturbance is identified, proper therapy can be initiated.

Fast Heart Rates:
Symptoms Beyond Palpitations

A fast heart rate can produce symptoms other than palpitations that can be very serious. An excessive rate puts a stress on the heart, forcing it to work much harder than usual. The heart muscle requires great amounts of fuel to perform this extra work. Patients with atherosclerotic coronary artery disease (blocked arteries in the heart) may be unable to deliver the required amounts, resulting in a fuel imbalance and the symptom of chest pain, which we call angina.

When patients with coronary artery disease develop angina during exertion, they can stop and rest, permitting the heart rate to slow down. However, most episodes of tachycardia are unrelated to the patient's activity level. The increase of the heart rate often occurs while the patient is at rest, and will not slow down by merely relaxing. The angina, likewise, will not go away until the heart rate slows down; this may require the use of drugs or an electrical shock.

Harvey C., a seventy-two-year-old man, experienced occasional attacks of angina ever since he had suffered a small heart attack two years earlier. One morning he abruptly, and unexpectedly, developed palpitations, and soon afterward complained of severe chest pain. Harvey went immediately to the nearest emergency room, thinking he was experiencing another heart attack.

The EKG revealed that his heart rate was extremely rapid (160 beats per minute) and irregular (a form of tachycardia, called atrial fibrillation). Atrial fibrillation is usually considered a stable heart rhythm because it does not degenerate into ventricular fibrillation and sudden death. However, it was pushing Harvey's heart rate too high.

Because he continued to feel poorly, and because his EKG

was demonstrating signs of cardiac stress, Harvey was given an intravenous sedative. After falling asleep almost immediately, he was administered a single electric shock to the chest wall, which succeeded in ending the tachycardia.

When Harvey awoke his chest pain was gone and his EKG returned to normal. He did not have a heart attack. Harvey spent two days in the hospital "for observation," then went home.

Harvey had a tachycardia that forced his heart up to an excessive and stressful rate (160 beats per minute). This created palpitations and severe angina, which could only be resolved when the tachycardia ended.

Tachycardias can push the heart to even faster rates. At rates greater than 250 beats per minute (which is very rare), the heart muscle demands tremendous amounts of blood, so that even normal arteries (those without atherosclerotic blockages) may be unable to deliver enough blood. These rapid heart rates can be very dangerous in otherwise healthy people, because even a healthy heart can't work this fast.

An additional danger results from the difficulty the heart has pumping blood at rapid heart rates. With increasing speed the heart becomes less efficient in sending blood to the rest of the body. When the heart beats at 120 beats per minute it has the potential to deliver twice as much blood to the rest of the body than when it beats at 60 beats per minute since then it is beating twice as fast. However, when the rate is 240 beats per minute it becomes less effective, because the heart is beating too quickly to fill up with blood properly. So even though the heart is beating quickly, it is not sending much blood to the rest of the body with each beat. This can cause the blood pressure to fall, which can result in fainting, shock, or even sudden death.

Gail L., a forty-two-year-old woman, went to the emergency room with a heart rate of 250 beats per minute, complaining of dizziness. She was found to have a markedly depressed blood pressure (70/30).

After being sedated, Gail was administered a single shock of electricity, returning her rhythm to normal, with a heart rate of 72 beats per minute and a blood pressure of 120/70 (which was her normal value).

There are only a handful of conditions that result in tachycardias as rapid as 240 beats per minute. At this very rapid heart rate Gail's heart could not fill adequately with blood. So, even though she had many heartbeats, each one pushed very little blood forward, resulting in a very low blood pressure. This becomes a medical emergency.

Very fast heart rates are serious because of the danger to the heart muscle (it may not get enough oxygen to do its work) and because the pump becomes inefficient, potentially causing a dangerous fall in blood pressure. Other forms of tachycardia have the potential to degenerate electrically into ventricular fibrillation: a transition from rapid (but organized) electrical stimulation to complete chaos resulting in sudden death.

A tachycardia usually comes and goes spontaneously. But once a tachycardia begins, it has the potential to continue indefinitely. If it does, we call it a sustained tachycardia, which then requires either medication or electricity to terminate. If the tachycardia is causing symptoms, then it may be urgent to treat immediately. Certain forms of tachycardia are well tolerated for long periods of time, and can even be treated at home with medications.

When tachycardias occur as short bursts (lasting for only seconds to minutes) we call them non-sustained. In these cases, drugs are required to suppress the return of the tachycardia. Although a non-sustained tachycardia may cause severe symptoms, the sustained forms are more likely to create trouble because they last longer.

Two Basic Types of Tachycardia

There are two basic types of tachycardia: 1. ventricular tachycardia (originating in the lower portion of the heart, called the ventricle), which is usually a very dangerous type; and 2. supraventricular tachycardia (originating *above* the ventricle, usually in the upper chambers, called the atria), which is typically more benign.

VENTRICULAR TACHYCARDIA
Ventricular tachycardia is the more dangerous form of tachycardia. It commonly degenerates to ventricular fibrillation and sudden death. In fact, most episodes of sudden death are preceded by ventricular tachycardia.

Even if it does not degenerate into ventricular fibrillation, ventricular tachycardia is poorly tolerated. The rates are often very rapid (ranging as high as 180 to 250 beats per minute), and the blood pressure frequently falls during an acute episode.

Seth L., a fifty-seven-year-old construction worker, had a heart attack. He recovered well, and had been without symptoms until one day, five years later, while carrying a box of supplies at work, he suddenly collapsed and was unconscious. Seth hit his head on a metal beam, requiring ten stitches to close the wound.

In the hospital he was found to have short "bursts" of ventricular tachycardia on his monitor (lasting from five to ten seconds).

It is likely that Seth had passed out because of a more prolonged episode of ventricular tachycardia lasting long enough to cause his blood pressure to fall significantly. He did not have another heart attack.

Seth had ventricular tachycardia because of the scar tissue left over from his *old* heart attack. Scar tissue can cause electrical instability in the heart many years after the attack, and can even result in sudden death. Seth was lucky not to have experienced ventricular fibrillation.

Seth was treated with drugs to suppress his ventricular tachycardia, and was sent home and back to work. He never again experienced a problem with dizziness or passing out.

Ventricular tachycardia usually occurs in people who have a diseased heart. Although the underlying heart problem may be serious, the presence of ventricular tachycardia worsens the prognosis.

There is a debate in the medical community about how (and even *if*) to treat ventricular tachycardia. Some doctors treat all cases immediately with medications. However, the drugs that are available can act unpredictably in these patients. Although we hope thereby to eliminate the electrical disturbance in the heart, any given medication has the potential to worsen the arrhythmia. Thus, when patients are administered a new drug, they must be carefully monitored.

Other scientists, taking a more aggressive position, suggest that medications should always be proven successful in the hospital, by electrical (EPS) testing of the heart (the same test given to sudden death survivors). Although the test is considered invasive, it can eliminate the guesswork from the final drug choice.

At the other end of the spectrum, many physicians will not treat ventricular tachycardia unless it is responsible for symptoms, such as severe palpitations, fainting, or chest pain.

Patients without symptoms can't feel better with therapy.

Although we would like to prevent sudden death, medications, which also have the potential to worsen the electrical stability of the heart have not been demonstrated to fulfill this goal.

George V., a seventy-eight-year-old man who had suffered a large heart attack five years earlier, was relatively active and had been feeling well. During a routine physical examination, however, he was found to have an irregular pulse. A twenty-four-hour cardiac monitor revealed multiple, short episodes of ventricular tachycardia.

The presence of episodic ventricular tachycardia indicates that George has a poor prognosis, which is unlikely to improve with medications. The arrhythmia is a reflection of severe muscular damage, which will remain severe after drug therapy. And George will not feel better, because he was otherwise unaware of the ventricular tachycardia.

Although many doctors would place George on medications, this course is not required. Because the drugs are expensive, have side effects, and have no proven benefit, many cardiologists would not treat George.

In contrast, sustained ventricular tachycardia is a medical emergency. A prolonged episode is usually poorly tolerated, resulting in a low blood pressure, dizziness, and chest pain, and it can degenerate into ventricular fibrillation and sudden death. A sustained episode usually requires an electric shock with the defibrillator to be converted back to normal.

While ventricular fibrillation requires a large amount of electricity (300 watt-seconds), ventricular tachycardia requires very little (20 watt-seconds) to return to normal. Even a thump on the chest might be adequate.

A sharp blow to the chest wall generates a small amount of natural electricity inside the chest. This can be enough to convert ventricular tachycardia back to normal sinus rhythm. However, a thump has the potential to destabilize the electrical rhythm. In rare cases it has converted ventricular tachycardia (a bad rhythm) into ventricular fibrillation (sudden death). It is recommended that an electric defibrillator be nearby when performing this maneuver.

SUPRAVENTRICULAR TACHYCARDIA (SVTS)

This is an entire family of tachycardias, all of which originate physically in the heart above the ventricles. They tend to be more benign than ventricular tachycardia because: 1. they do not usually degenerate into ventricular fibrillation and sudden death; and 2. they tend to be slower, and more easily tolerated.

These arrhythmias can occur without symptoms or patient awareness and might be discovered only during a medical examination. In other patients, they can cause symptoms that range from palpitations to chest pain. SVTs can even result in cardiac arrest and death, but this is very uncommon.

There are several types of SVT, with different features to their clinical symptoms and therapy:

1. *Sinus tachycardia:* This is the normal increase in heart rate caused by exercise or activity, regulated by the sinus node (the body's natural pacemaker). This does not require therapy.

2. *Atrial tachycardia:* Although the sinus node is the natural pacemaker, other parts of the heart can take control of the heart rate. Certain cells in the atria are capable of generating rapid electrical signals (as fast as 180 beats per minute).

Atrial tachycardia is very common, even among young adults. In fact, many of us have very short bursts of this arrhythmia while we sleep (a situation that is completely benign, and does not require treatment). Those who have episodes while awake often experience palpitations, chest pain, and even light-headedness. In these cases medications are required.

3. *Atrial fibrillation/atrial flutter:* These two conditions are characterized by extremely rapid impulses generated in the atria (flutter is usually 300 beats per minute; fibrillation is usually greater than 350 beats per minute). But the main pumps of the heart (the ventricles) cannot tolerate beating at these excessive rates. Fortunately, the heart has a safety device called the A-V node, which protects the ventricles by blocking many of the rapid beats. Each beat must pass through the A-V node in order to travel from the atria to the ventricles. These conditions can cause the same symptoms as atrial tachycardia, and generally require therapy.

Slow Heart Rates

The electrical system can break down, causing the heart to beat too slowly, or to stop altogether. Problems can occur anywhere along its extensive network.

The sinus node is a collection of very special cells that sit in a corner of the heart and regulate the heart rate. These cells repeatedly generate electrical impulses. When the heart must beat faster (for example, during exercise), the sinus node generates the impulses at a faster rate. Each of these signals produces one heartbeat. We say the heart is in "normal sinus rhythm" when the electrical system is working normally.

The impulse from the sinus node spreads via natural wires throughout the upper chambers of the heart (the atria), causing

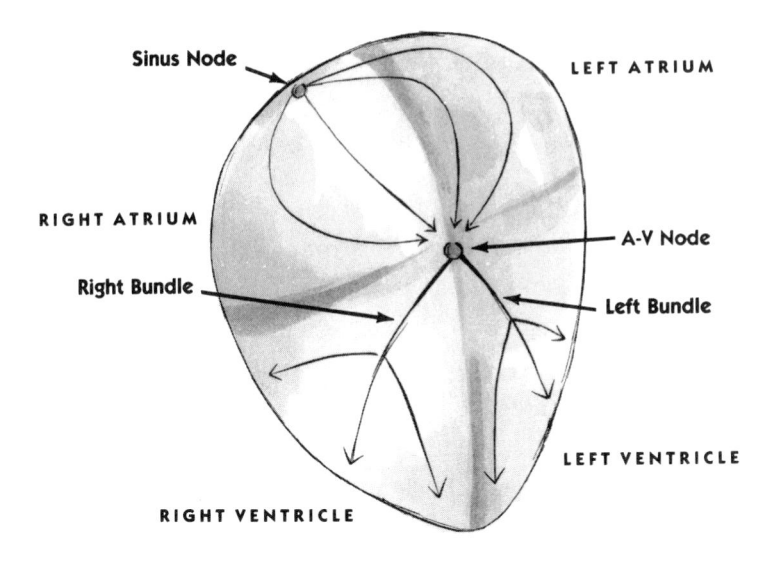

Electrical system of the heart

the chambers to contract. The electricity then converges on the A-V node (atrio-ventricular node), which is an electrical relay station between the atria and the ventricles. Every impulse must pass through this special group of cells before reaching the main pumps (the ventricles). As mentioned before, it protects the ventricles from excessive rates.

The A-V node sends the electrical impulse forward to the ventricles through two major pathways, called the "right bundle" and the "left bundle," which further divide into smaller branches.

Damage to the sinus node, A-V node (the relay station), or the natural wires can slow down, or even stop, the flow of electricity in the heart. If the heart beats too slowly, the amount of blood sent to the rest of the body including the brain can be seriously diminished. This can result in light-headedness and fainting.

Karen H., an eighty-two-year-old woman, was in the kitchen, talking on the phone with her daughter, when she suddenly fell over. She had no warning before she fell (some people feel light-headed first). Karen broke her hip as a result of the fall.

In the hospital it was discovered that Karen had a very slow pulse (averaging 40 beats per minute). In addition, Karen was observed on the monitor to have an episode in which her heart did not beat for four seconds. A pacemaker was recommended.

This is a common story. Karen fell *because* of the slowing of her heartbeat. A heart rate of 40 beats per minute is too slow for a person this age. The rate is not fast enough to deliver enough blood to the body for all of its activities. A well-trained athlete might manage with a pulse slower than 50 beats per minute, but an eighty-two-year-old woman needs a greater heart rate.

More important, the presence of a pause (longer than three seconds) is considered serious in anyone who has fainted. In Karen's example, she had a four-second pause. During those four seconds her heart was *not* pumping any blood. As a result, her blood pressure certainly experienced a significant fall, which explains why Karen lost consciousness.

Karen had deterioration of her sinus node, resulting in slow heart rate and long pauses. This is a common problem with the aging although it certainly does not affect everybody. For unknown reasons, scar tissue is formed within the electrical system, affecting either the natural pacemaker (sinus node) or the conduction system. The end result is to block the generation and/or transmission of electrical impulses to the heart muscle.

The electrical system usually does not abruptly stop working (if it did, this would result in sudden death). Instead, most people have short moments of failure, followed by the rapid return of electrical impulses. The severity of symptoms depends on how long the system shuts down.

Without an electric signal, the heart will not beat. This can result in a moment of light-headedness (if the pause is a short one), overt fainting (with a longer pause, as with Karen), or sudden death (if the heart does not start again after the pause).

This breakdown of the electrical system can affect people of all ages. Although it is more common in people of advanced age, there are occasional examples of men and women in their twenties and thirties with sinus-node and conduction-system disease.

A heart attack can abruptly interrupt the electrical system. The sinus node, A-V node, and the conduction system are all made up of living cells. If these cells are deprived of their blood supply they will die. As a result, some heart attacks (those involving the arteries supplying these special cells) will result in slowed or interrupted electrical transmission.

When electrical problems are serious, regardless of the underlying cause, the cure is a pacemaker.

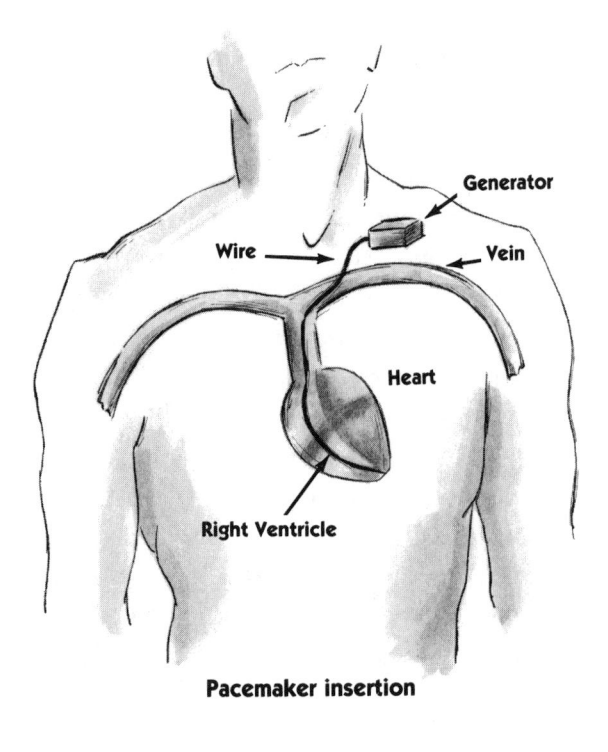

Generator

Wire

Vein

Heart

Right Ventricle

Pacemaker insertion

Myth #3:
"My life will be ruined if I need a pacemaker!"

This is a common but unfounded fear. A pacemaker *improves* the quality of one's life, it does not worsen it. Once placed, it allows the patient to resume physical activities that would otherwise have been a problem. Many people who receive pacemakers had been passing out, or experiencing fatigue because of a low heart rate. Some are at higher risk for sudden death without the pacemaker.

A pacemaker is a surgically implanted device that generates electrical impulses through a small generator and sends them to the heart through a small wire. If there is a failure of the sinus node (the natural pacemaker) or an interruption in the conduction system, an artificial pacemaker can fix the problem. The pacemaker wire is placed below the blockage in the electrical system, so that an impulse can still reach the heart muscle.

The operation to insert a pacemaker is relatively minor. The generator is implanted under the skin of the chest, just beneath the collarbone. The wire is inserted through a vein, and is "threaded" in the direction of blood flow to the inside of the right ventricle. The impulse from the pacemaker first stimulates the right ventricle, then spreads to the rest of the heart muscle, allowing it to beat.

People who have pacemakers are totally unaware of the pacemaker's presence as it performs its work. They do not feel any shock from the pacemaker, because the electrical impulse is of very low amplitude. It is just enough to stimulate the heart to beat.

People with pacemakers may shower, swim, run, engage in sexual activity, and are even allowed to be in a room with a microwave oven. This last fear was the result of a real, but now outdated, problem. Pacemakers have sophisticated electronic memories that can be altered by magnetic waves. Older microwave ovens were built with very poor shielding, and had the potential to interfere with the memory circuits of a pacemaker. But better shielding of both microwave ovens and pacemakers has made this possibility extremely unlikely. Although we still warn people with pacemakers to avoid unnecessary exposure to devices that emit high energy, this is not a major problem.

Most pacemakers are programmed to generate an impulse only when the heart fails to do so by itself. If, for example, a pacemaker is "set" for a heart rate of 60 beats per minute, it will not generate any impulses while the natural heart rate is greater than 60 beats per minute. But if the heart rate falls below 60 beats per minute, the pacemaker will kick in. It will generate 60 electronic impulses every minute (at a rate of 1 every second) until the natural heart rate speeds up again. Pacemakers can be programmed for different rates. Although most are set at fixed rates, some can be programmed to increase their rate with an increase in the activity of the body, which is more physiologic. There are many models and types from which doctors can choose.

Pacemakers are powered by batteries, which can last for many years. They do eventually run out, in perhaps five to seven years. People with pacemakers are asked to have frequent checks of their battery and their pacemaker circuits. Today this can be done through a telephone directly to the doctor's office. The operation to change the battery (which involves changing the entire generator) is minor.

The generator, which lies directly under the skin, is removed surgically with local anesthesia. The wires, which run to the heart, are checked and are usually in good shape. The generator is replaced with a fresh one, which is attached to the old wires assuming they are intact.

Some pacemakers are unnecessarily inserted. In fact, in 1983 a group of specialists in a large metropolitan area reviewed the indications for pacemaker insertion.[1] They concluded that 44 percent were definitely indicated, 36 percent were possibly indicated, and 20 percent were not indicated. When considering that there are 120,000 pacemakers implanted every year in the United States, a large number may be implanted unnecessarily.

Some patients have absolute indications for a permanent artificial pacemaker, like Karen H., who had fainted with a very low heart rate. There are very specific guidelines available to doctors that evaluate the absolute versus the relative need for a pacemaker. It is always reasonable to get a second opinion if one is prescribed by your doctor.

Some people have less serious problems with their conduction system. Although the electrocardiogram is abnormal in these cases, the condition is not necessarily clinically important.

For example, it is relatively common for people to develop a block in one of the major wires that carry electrical signals throughout the ventricles (the right or left bundle). When this occurs, the electric signal can reach the ventricles through the other, healthy bundle. Although the impulse does not spread evenly through the ventricles (because it travels down only one of the bundles), the pumps will function normally. The EKG will detect this abnormal spread of electricity.

If *both* bundles were to become completely blocked, then there would be no means for the electric signal to reach the ventricles. Thus, when one bundle is blocked, the other one must be watched carefully. If it shows early signs of trouble, a pacemaker would be indicated.

∧∧∧∧∧

CHAPTER EIGHT

Heart Murmurs

There is something a little scary about having a "heart murmur," which is misunderstood by most people. Some think that a murmur is an arrhythmia or a skipped beat in the heart. Others think it means the heart is weak. But most simply don't know.

A heart murmur is merely any sound made by blood flowing through the heart. For some people a murmur reflects a serious problem with the heart: those who have rheumatic heart disease, narrowed valves, and leaky valves. In others, a murmur has absolutely no clinical importance. Most people who were told that they had a heart murmur in their childhood had (and have) absolutely nothing wrong with them.

"Mitral valve prolapse" (which commonly causes a heart murmur) is a condition that has assumed an importance out of proportion to its true significance. The majority of people with mitral valve prolapse (there are millions) are totally healthy. Unfortunately, many of these patients think that they have a heart condition, and require reassurance. A small number of people have a serious form of mitral valve prolapse, and they require special observation and therapy. But most people do not have to worry.

There are many misconceptions about the need and use of antibiotics in patients with valvular disease, mitral valve prolapse, and in those with simple heart murmurs. We will explore all these issues as we explore murmurs, the heart, and its valves.

Myth #1:
A heart murmur is always serious. If you have a heart murmur, you have a problem with your heart.

Although heart murmurs can certainly *reflect* a serious problem with the heart, most are totally benign.

Kevin H., an eighteen-year-old man, went for a routine physical examination before going to college. He was nervous about going for the checkup, but things were going surprisingly well, until the doctor listened over Kevin's chest with the stethoscope.

After several minutes of listening, the doctor looked up and said, "You have a heart murmur. I don't think it's anything important, but I'm going to send you to a specialist to be sure."

Kevin was convinced that he had a serious problem with his heart. He fantasized that he would need an operation, or maybe that he would die. He remembered that he recently felt some chest pain after playing football with his friends and wondered if he did anything wrong by not having seen a doctor earlier.

Anxiously, Kevin went to the heart specialist three weeks later. He was examined by the doctor, and had several tests of his heart. The doctor reported, "Everything is normal. You have what we call a 'functional murmur.' It means nothing. You and your heart are totally healthy!"

Kevin was relieved. His bill for the visit was $850 ($250 for the doctor, and $600 for the tests).

This is a common scenario. A patient with a murmur is often sent to a cardiologist for evaluation. Yet many of these people have nothing wrong with them. This is especially common among pregnant women.

Virtually every pregnant woman will develop a heart murmur because of the increase of maternal blood flow that is associated with a normal, healthy pregnancy. Although this murmur is totally normal (and is even expected), many pregnant women are sent to internists and cardiologists for evaluation. Only a small number are discovered to have an important problem with the heart. The majority of pregnant women who have a significant cardiac condition know about their problem before their pregnancy.

A murmur can be either "functional" (which is clinically unimportant) or more serious, reflecting true heart disease. Yet, regardless of clinical importance, murmurs are defined as follows: *any sound (heard with a stethoscope) that is caused by the flow of blood through the heart*.

Blood usually moves quietly through the chambers of the heart. With each beat the heart muscle squeezes down, ejecting blood through its valves from chamber to chamber and into the aorta (for delivery to the rest of the body). As blood is ejected out of the heart it makes a soft sound: usually too soft to be heard with the stethoscope.

But under certain conditions the flow of blood through the heart can be heard. If otherwise normal flow is increased or exaggerated (such as during exercise), a sound will be heard as the blood is ejected from the heart and is called a functional, ejection, or flow murmur.

On the other hand, if the heart has an internal abnormality, such as a diseased valve, the flow of blood becomes distorted, creating a loud sound also called a murmur. In cases like this, the murmur is not the problem, but a *reflection* of the disease within the heart. In contrast, a functional murmur does not reflect an underlying problem because it is an exaggeration of a normal event.

There are two distinct phases to every heartbeat: when the heart is squeezing down, pushing blood forward (called systole); and when the heart is relaxing, and filling with blood (called diastole). A murmur can be heard during either of these two phases, because blood is flowing during both, either in or out of the heart.

By listening with the stethoscope, a doctor can tell whether a murmur occurs during systole or diastole, which helps to define what is wrong with the heart. Each type of murmur can be defined by special characteristics (timing, pitch, and duration) that help to identify the underlying cardiac problem. With each heartbeat comes a new cycle of emptying (systole) and filling (diastole), and thus the murmur is constantly repeated.

Functional (or ejection) murmurs occur during systole, when blood is ejected out of the heart. They are common, occurring anytime that blood flow is exaggerated, and do not reflect any underlying heart disease. They are frequently heard in:

1. People who are thin. If the chest is thin, the heart is closer to the stethoscope, and all sounds are exaggerated. It is easier to hear a flow murmur in children because of their small size.

2. People with athletic hearts. Athletes typically have an increased flow of blood through their hearts with each beat

(they are better conditioned). Thus, a flow murmur is more likely to be heard.

3. Pregnant women. During pregnancy the mother's body produces extra blood to help nurture the fetus, causing the mother's blood volume to expand. The heart, therefore, pumps more blood because there is more to pump. This increased activity creates a flow murmur.

These flow murmurs do not reflect problems with the heart. Yet people with flow murmurs are often sent to cardiologists for evaluation. A careful examination can usually distinguish an innocent flow murmur from a more serious murmur. There is an increased reliance on medical technology to validate the clinical impression that everything is "okay."

The echocardiogram is a safe and easy test that can demonstrate what the physical examination suggests—that a murmur is either benign, or that there is significant heart disease.

ECHOCARDIOGRAM

This test (also called an ECHO test, or cardiac sonogram) involves placing a round device (called a transducer) on the chest, transmitting sound waves to the heart and measuring the reflection. Sections of the heart closer to the machine bounce the waves more quickly to the machine. A computer, using this information, constructs an image of the heart, allowing the doctor to visualize the size and strength of the heart muscle and to examine the structure of the heart valves. A more sophisticated ECHO machine (called a Doppler) can, additionally, measure the flow of blood through the heart valves.

The ECHO test is risk-free because it does not require needles, does not use radiation, and the sound waves are harmless. Although the test is safe, it is somewhat expensive, and there may be too great a reliance on its performance. A good physical examination can answer most clinical questions, and can certainly reveal the presence of serious valvular heart disease.

Myth #2:
"If I have a normal ECHO *test, I will not have a heart attack."*

This is a common assumption. Many patients, when told that the ECHO is normal, feel reassured. But they misunderstand the purpose of the test. The ECHO provides no direct information about the coronary arteries. The test can demonstrate muscle damage from an old or new heart attack. But it cannot anticipate whether there will be cardiologic events in the future.

The ECHO is extremely valuable in defining the function of the heart valves. If a patient with a murmur has a normal ECHO, then it is likely that it is functional.

Sometimes a murmur is not so innocent. If the internal structure of the heart is abnormal, the flow of blood will typically be turbulent. This abnormal flow of blood is also heard by the stethoscope as a murmur, which, in this case, reflects disease of the heart. It is usually easy to separate the functional flow murmurs from more serious murmurs.

Many different problems, mainly those of the heart valves, produce abnormal murmurs. The valves are central to the flow of blood. Each of the four chambers of the heart has a valve through which all blood must pass. The valves are vital because they ensure that blood will flow in only one direction through the heart by allowing blood to leave, but not to return.

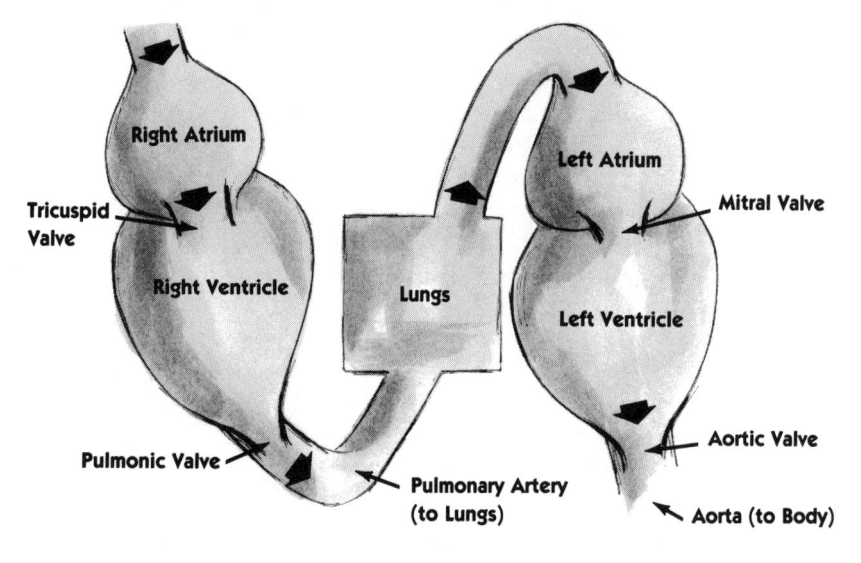

Schematic diagram of heart: Four chambers and four valves

Blood flows through the four chambers (and their valves) as follows:

1. Blood in the right atrium is ejected through the *tricuspid valve* and enters the right ventricle.

2. Blood in the right ventricle is ejected through the *pulmonic valve* into the pulmonic artery where it enters the lungs. The blood picks up oxygen while it is in the lungs. Blood then flows into the left atrium.

3. Blood in the left atrium is ejected through the *mitral valve* and enters the left ventricle.

4. Blood in the left ventricle is ejected through the *aortic valve* and enters the aorta, and is then sent to the rest of the body.

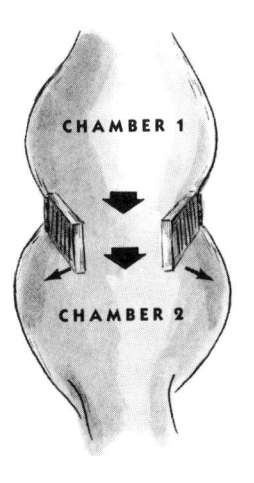 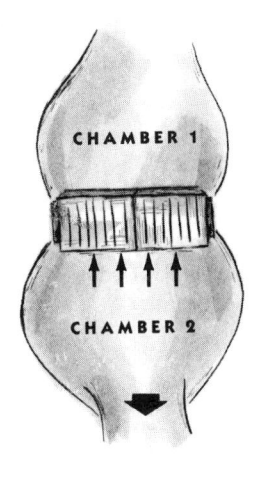

Normal valve: Saloon doors opening and closing

Blood must pass through each of the four valves as it travels through the heart, and any change in the structure of the heart valves will change the mechanics of blood flow resulting in a murmur.

The heart valves are similar to saloon doors (as in old western movies). When a chamber of the heart squeezes down, blood is ejected forward, pushing open the swinging doors of the valve as it moves into the next chamber. After filling with blood, this next chamber will in turn squeeze down, continuing to push the blood forward.

The heart valves are one-way doors that prevent blood from returning into the first chamber when the second chamber contracts. When the second chamber squeezes down, the doors shut tight. They do not allow blood to travel backward, because they do not swing back in the *opposite* direction. The blood can only move forward.

Thus, heart valves have two functions. They must open to allow blood to move forward, and they must close to prevent

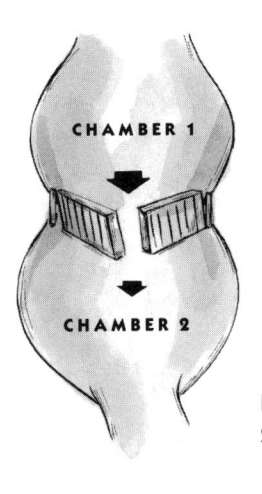

Narrowed valve:
Saloon doors with rusty hinges

blood from moving backward. Therefore there are two types of problems that can occur with these valves: 1. they can fail to open normally (limiting the forward flow of blood); or 2. they can fail to close normally (permitting the backward flow of blood).

Both problems, although very different from each other, can be very serious. Both cause turbulent blood flow and produce murmurs. But more important, both can interfere with the normal function of the heart, causing a variety of symptoms (chest pain, shortness of breath, fatigue, fainting spells) and potentially causing sudden death.

Failure to Open Normally (Stenosis)

Valves can narrow (medically called stenosis) and fail to open normally, limiting the amount of forward blood flow. This is analogous to the saloon doors with rusty hinges, opening only partially.

Once a cycle of damage begins, the heart valves become progressively more damaged and narrowed, and the patient becomes sicker and sicker.

Valves narrow for different reasons. It can merely be the consequence of aging. Over the years calcium from the blood can deposit on the surface of the valves. The process can continue until, eventually, a valve has become critically narrowed. Although we do not understand why only *some* patients develop calcium deposits, wear and tear of the valves can accelerate this process.

Valves can become damaged by the body's own defense system, which is responsible for releasing a series of toxic and erosive chemicals when it detects an invading infectious organism. Besides fighting the infection, these chemicals can also seriously damage the body as well, a condition called inflammation.

Inflammation causes swelling, redness, and pain in the body and often results in the formation of scar tissue, which is part of healing. When this occurs in the heart, the valves begin to thicken and eventually have difficulty opening.

Rheumatic fever is an important cause of inflammation of heart valves, and is often responsible for their narrowing. Although many people have heard of rheumatic fever, most are confused about what it actually is.

Myth #3:
"I had rheumatic fever as a child."

Although some people *did* have rheumatic fever when they were young, many who think (and were told) that they did actually did not. There was a time when a child who had fever and a heart murmur was automatically assumed to have rheumatic fever. Often these children were told that they could not play with other kids and could not participate in the usual physical activities because their parents were afraid that their child had a weak heart. Many of these children were limited for no reason. The diagnosis of rheumatic fever was grossly overused.

Rheumatic fever is a specific diagnosis. It is an illness with very specific consequences to the body (mainly to the heart). Its diagnosis cannot be made casually. There are some very rigorous criteria that must be satisfied to confirm the diagnosis of acute rheumatic fever.

Rheumatic fever is not, itself, an infection. Instead, it is a chain reaction involving the body's immune system which occurs several weeks after healing from a strep throat infection. Although the infection occurred in the throat, the resultant immune reaction occurs in the heart.

There are many types of throat infections, most of which are viral. Those called strep throats (common in children) involve a specific bacterium, called streptococcus. Antibiotics easily eliminate this infection, but if it is not promptly treated, the body can develop a terrible reaction.

Without the help of antibiotics, the patient's body starts to create antibodies to fight the bacteria: tiny bullets that attack the invading organisms. After the body studies the invader, it produces antibodies specifically designed to fight the particular infection.

With streptococcal throat infection, a very unusual reaction can occur. In order to protect itself, the streptococcus organism has evolved over the years to disguise itself from the body's immune system. The bacteria attempt to escape attack by tricking the immune system into thinking that they belong in the body. The bacteria's outer chemical structure resembles the outer chemical structure of the heart.

A serious thing can occur due to this similarity. The immune system eventually starts to make antibodies to the bacteria. When the antibodies are finally released, they attack both the bacteria *and* the patient's own heart. The antibodies, designed to recognize the bacteria, are confused and believe that the heart is one of the invading organisms.

The heart is attacked, resulting in a serious (and potentially fatal) illness called acute rheumatic fever. It occurs, on average, from ten days to two weeks after the throat infection. The illness is characterized by fever, a rash, a heart murmur, weakness of the heart, arthritis (joints are also attacked), and even brain involvement. Antibiotics are useless at this stage, because the original infection is already gone. The attack comes from the body's own immune system.

An attack of acute rheumatic fever can last up to three months. The body continues to make antibodies, because it still thinks that the heart is an invading organism. Sad to report, even when a patient passes the acute episode (which can sometimes even cause death), the victim's problems are not necessarily over. In more than half of these patients, a chain reaction has begun, and the damage continues slowly in the heart for years.

One to two decades later (on average, twelve years after the initial attack of rheumatic fever), this results in serious injury to the valves of the heart. Although each of the four valves can be affected, the mitral valve is almost always the first to become damaged. In fact, rheumatic fever is essentially the only known cause of mitral stenosis (the narrowing of the mitral valve).

Rheumatic fever can be effectively prevented if the strep throat is treated promptly with antibiotics. Even without treatment it is still difficult to contract rheumatic fever. But avoiding antibiotics places a person at an unnecessary risk. Because of the widespread availability of penicillin, rheumatic fever is no longer very common in the United States. Yet it still occurs in great numbers in underdeveloped countries and among more indigent Americans.

Thus the inflammation of rheumatic fever, and aging (with the deposits of calcium) both can cause stenosis of heart valves. But, regardless of the mechanism of stenosis, the net effect is to limit the amount of blood that travels through the heart. In the most serious cases, an operation is required.

Though each of the four valves can develop stenosis, the two valves on the left side of the heart (the mitral valve and the aortic valve) more commonly develop this problem. And each has its own characteristic clinical findings when they become narrowed.

MITRAL STENOSIS

Almost exclusively the consequence of rheumatic fever, the narrowing of this valve will obstruct the flow of blood into the left ventricle. A normal mitral valve, while it is wide open, allows for more than enough blood to freely enter the left ventricle from the left atrium. Mitral stenosis can markedly reduce the size of the open valve and limit blood flow. It is considered critically narrowed when the valve opening is less than 20 percent of the original area.

A valve this critically narrowed requires surgical repair. These patients tend to be very sick, and surgical repair can dramatically improve their symptoms and level of day-to-day function.

A characteristic murmur can usually be heard in people with mitral stenosis. As the blood struggles to enter the left ventricle, it fights its way through the narrowed valve and makes turbulence, just as water rushes more loudly through a garden hose after pinching the end, near the nozzle.

The murmur from the turbulence occurs during diastole—

the period of time when the left ventricle is filling with blood from the left atrium, through the mitral valve. It is typically a soft, low-pitched rumbling noise and has been compared to the sound made by a wagon rolling over a wooden bridge in the distance. Although it often takes some experience to recognize, it is a very distinct murmur, and its presence during a physical exam is usually enough to diagnose mitral stenosis.

By slowing the rate at which blood passes through, mitral stenosis results in a backup of blood. Pressure builds up in the left atrium, which in turn is transmitted back to the lungs. This leads to congestion, which results in a feeling of shortness of breath, the most common symptom of mitral stenosis.

This can be a significant symptom (some people are unable to climb a flight of stairs or walk a single block because of shortness of breath). If the symptoms become this severe, the patient needs to have the valve fixed. There are no medicines that can do this. There are no drugs capable of opening up a narrowed valve. There are two surgical options: the valve can be repaired or replaced.

In cases in which the valve can be repaired (called a val-vuloplasty), the surgeon opens the heart and cuts free the narrowed portions of the valve, analogous to loosening the hinges of the saloon doors, so that it can open more normally. This is the preferred method when it is technically possible because nothing artificial is put in the heart. Some valves are so seriously damaged that they can't be repaired, and hence require complete replacement.

Artificial valves are not as good as original, healthy valves. They have a serious potential for attracting blood clots and infections. But the cure is clearly better than the disease.

Most patients feel better after surgery, and many will live longer because of the valve replacement.

AORTIC STENOSIS

This is a very serious condition. The aortic valve is the final valve through which blood flows through the heart. The left ventricle must pump all blood through this valve in order to send blood to the rest of the body. When this valve becomes narrowed, there are very serious symptoms and consequences (including a serious risk of sudden death).

Rheumatic fever can cause the aortic valve to narrow. But this is not a common cause of aortic stenosis. The two most important causes are: 1. an abnormal valve from birth; and 2. the deposits of calcium with age.

Up to 1 percent of all people are born with an abnormally shaped aortic valve, which can cause difficulty later in life. A normal aortic valve has three small cusps which are like three little swinging doors. In contrast, some people are born with valves that have two larger cusps.

Having a bicuspid valve (with two cusps) is usually not a serious problem. In fact, most people with this abnormality do not know for most of their lives that anything is wrong. The valve can work normally for many years, but the abnormal shape makes these valves vulnerable. They tend to stiffen and to narrow with age. This is the result of increased stress on the valve. A normal valve with three doors has less stress on each door than a valve with only two doors.

Nearly 10 percent of people with bicuspid valves will get into serious trouble and develop a significant stenosis. The problem is progressive. Once the valve begins to narrow, the condition continues to worsen to the point of requiring surgical correction. Surgery is usually necessary before these patients turn sixty years old, but it is sometimes needed in those as young as forty or fifty years of age.

A more serious birth defect occurs when the aortic valve is formed with only one very large cusp. This type of aortic valve is called unicuspid and it does not work well at all, causing clinical problems almost immediately after birth. Most children with unicuspid aortic valves require surgical repair before they are one year old. Fortunately, this is a rare condition. As with bicuspid aortic valves, the problem occurs during fetal development.

People with normal (tricuspid) aortic valves can also develop serious stiffening and narrowing of their valves. The usual wear and tear of life can lead to the slow but steady deposit of calcium onto a normal aortic valve with advancing age. It usually first becomes noticeable in people older than sixty-five (most commonly in patients in their seventies and eighties).

People with bicuspid aortic valves typically get into trouble at younger ages than those with tricuspid valves (although there are always exceptions to the rule). Regardless of the cause or age of onset, aortic stenosis can be a very serious problem.

The murmur of aortic stenosis reflects the struggle of blood to leave the left ventricle (with mitral stenosis the murmur occurs as blood enters this chamber). This causes a high-pitched blowing sound, occurring during systole, the period of left ventricular contraction and emptying. Although it can sometimes be confused with the benign ejection murmur (both occur during the ejection of blood out of the heart), the murmur of aortic stenosis reflects an obstruction to the flow of blood out of the heart. An ejection murmur, in contrast, occurs because of exaggerated blood flow out of the heart.

Aortic stenosis can be detected in other ways during a physical examination. Feeling the pulse of an artery is a helpful clue. Normally, blood bounds through arteries, making the pulse feel strong and brisk. But with aortic stenosis the blood is hung up. The exit is too small and the heart strains in its effort to get the blood out. This makes the pulse feel weak and drawn out. A weakened pulse can help to separate people who have significant aortic stenosis from those who have only a benign ejection murmur.

Aortic stenosis can cause some very serious symptoms. The most important of these include fainting, chest pain with physical activity, and shortness of breath. These symptoms can interrupt and limit a person's activities. But, equally important, they are also a very serious warning that sudden death may be around the corner.

The life expectancy of a patient with aortic stenosis is significantly reduced once these symptoms begin. Those who feel chest pain have less than a 50 percent chance of living five years, and those with shortness of breath have less than a two-year life expectancy.

Open-heart surgery can help these patients. Replacing the heart valve with an artificial valve eliminates most of the symptoms and certainly reduces the risk of sudden death. The new valve allows blood to flow more freely out of the heart, relieving the stress on the heart. As with mitral stenosis, drugs can't effectively treat this condition. Although they can help reduce some of the symptoms, ultimately the valve needs to be physically repaired.

In contrast, those people with aortic stenosis who have no symptoms very rarely suffer from sudden death. The risk is less than 1 percent a year. Thus, if an abnormal valve is detected in an otherwise asymptomatic person, nothing need be done. The patient can be monitored by office visits and followed for the possible development of symptoms. Until that time there is no reason to fix the valve.

Valvuloplasty

An alternative to surgery, called balloon valvuloplasty, has become available in the past five years to fix narrowed heart valves. It is a technique by which a heart valve (mitral and/ or aortic) can be forced open with an inflatable balloon. Surgery is not required, and the patient is awake during the entire repair.

A cardiac catheterization is performed, and a plastic tube is advanced through the narrowed valve. A balloon which has been collapsed around the tube is inflated, and literally forces open the valve.

It is attractive to fix a heart valve without surgery, but this technique is hardly perfect. There is a 4 percent chance of a patient's dying during this procedure (actually less than the chance of dying during surgery for the oldest and sickest patients), and the valve is not as well repaired with the balloon as it would be through surgery.

The balloon will increase the size of the valve, on average, by only 50 percent, leaving the valve far from normal, although it is usually enough to reverse most symptoms. The artificial valve inserted during surgery is still smaller than a healthy, normal heart valve but it is significantly larger than the result after balloon repair.

Furthermore, re-stenosis is a significant problem with the balloon technique. Even when the procedure is initially a success, the valve inevitably becomes narrow again, sometimes within several weeks to months. In one scientific study, up to 50 percent of the dilated valves re-narrowed within eight months of the original procedure. Most of these patients required another dilation, or surgery. The surgical results last much longer, as there is no problem with re-stenosis after surgery.

Some patients are too sick and too old for valve surgery. If the risk of an operation is considered too great, the balloon valvuloplasty is a reasonable alternative. For otherwise young and strong people, surgery should be the first choice (even though it is more attractive to avoid the operation). The surgical benefits are extremely well established; those of the balloon technique remain uncertain.

"Leaky Valves"
(Insufficiency/Regurgitation)

In contrast to stenosis, in which a heart valve is unable to open normally, the failure of a valve to close normally is referred to as leaky (called either insufficiency or regurgitation in medical parlance).

Under normal circumstances, when a chamber of the heart contracts blood is pushed forward. The exit valve swings open. The previous valve through which blood had entered the chamber should swing shut allowing blood to travel only in the forward direction.

If a valve is leaky, it will not stay shut, and blood will be allowed to flow backward into the previous chamber. The leaky valve can be compared to the saloon doors swinging open in the opposite direction.

Doctors often use the term leaky heart valve, but it is a poor choice.

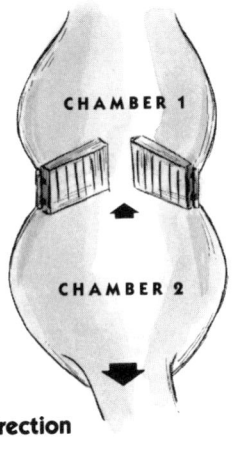

Leaky valve:
Saloon doors swing back in opposite direction

Myth #4:
If you have a "leaky" heart valve, blood is literally
leaking out of the heart.

Leaky is a charged word, evoking an image of a leaking faucet. One of my patients actually thought that he was slowly bleeding into his chest, from his heart, because one of his valves leaked. This is not the case. The term leaky is not a very good one. These diseased valves fail to shut normally, and fail to prevent the backflow of blood. Thus, the terms regurgitant and insufficient are more accurate.

Valves will become leaky or regurgitant if they are damaged in several different ways. In some, the valve is damaged by a bacterial infection, which we call *endocarditis* (infection of the heart valves). Bacteria will erode and make holes in the cusps of the valve. Blood is not held back even when the valve shuts closed, because it can leak through the holes in the valve.

Syphilis was once a very common cause for aortic regurgitation. This peculiar infection travels through the blood and eventually attacks different parts of the body, including the aortic valve. The damage to the valve is slow, and does not become clinically apparent until many years later. While it is not very common today because we are more successful at recognizing and effectively treating syphilis, sporadic cases are identified.

Some people have degeneration of their valves. With age their valves weaken physically because of a chemical change in the tissue itself. For reasons that are unclear, the usually firm valves soften and get floppy.

When shut closed, the weakened valves will stretch under the pressure. They eventually flip open in the opposite direction because of their softness. This results in leaking of the heart valve.

The degenerative process will occur only in some people. It will not happen to most of us. But tissue degeneration accounts for the majority of cases of those who develop heart-valve regurgitation.

All four valves of the heart can become regurgitant, but the valves on the left side of the heart (mitral and aortic) are more commonly involved, as with stenosis. But unlike stenosis (which is always a chronic condition), regurgitation can be either acute or chronic.

A heart valve does not narrow very quickly. All of the conditions that cause stenosis take years and years to evolve. Thus, the heart has time to make gradual adjustments. But in the long run the heart can't handle the stress.

Regurgitation, however, can be abrupt. An infection can turn an otherwise normal valve into a leaky valve within hours. When the process is sudden and acute, the heart has a difficult time dealing with the tremendous stress. As a result the patient becomes ill immediately and often surgery is required on an emergency basis.

Regurgitation can alternatively evolve slowly. The process of tissue degeneration usually occurs over a period of many years. In these cases the heart has time to make adjustments to the stress. In contrast, abrupt regurgitation does not allow the heart time to adjust.

Daniel J., a twenty-eight-year-old man, went for a routine physical examination although he was feeling totally well. Surprisingly his heart was found to be mildly enlarged, and a characteristic murmur of mitral regurgitation was heard by the physician.

Daniel underwent an echocardiogram, which revealed severe regurgitation of his mitral valve.

Because he has no symptoms, Daniel does not require any therapy at present. However, he will probably require a surgical valve replacement in the future because his heart will eventually feel the effects of this chronic stress.

In contrast:

Bruce T., a fifty-two-year-old man, had a small heart attack, which resulted in damage to his mitral valve, causing it to leak abruptly. An echocardiogram revealed a moderate amount of regurgitation (less than what Daniel J. experienced). Bruce became extremely ill, requiring placement on a respirator. He was rushed to surgery for valve replacement, and did very well afterward.

The difference between Daniel and Bruce is very important. Daniel had chronic mitral regurgitation, whereas in Bruce it was acute. Even though Daniel had more severe regurgitation of his mitral valve, he had no symptoms. Bruce, with less valvular disease, was critically ill because his heart had no time to adjust. Daniel had many years to accommodate the slow erosion of his valve.

The same amount of leaking has very different implications depending on its time of evolution for both aortic and mitral regurgitation. We quantify the amount of leaking of all heart valves on a scale of 0 + (no leaking) to 4 + (the most severe leaking). Although there are specific, and rigid, criteria available to quantify regurgitation on this scale, in essence 1 + is considered mild, 2 + and 3 + are considered moderate, and 4 + is severe regurgitation (for both the aortic and mitral valves).

MITRAL REGURGITATION

Normally, when the left ventricle squeezes down, blood is ejected out of the heart through the opened aortic valve and goes to the rest of the body. Blood can't travel backward, into the left atrium, because the mitral valve closes completely shut.

But when the mitral valve is regurgitant, it fails to close normally. This allows for backflow of blood into the left atrium when the left ventricle squeezes down. Blood flows in two directions, both forward and backward through the heart.

The characteristic murmur of mitral regurgitation occurs during systole, when the left ventricle contracts. It is typically high-pitched and very loud. In addition, the backflow of blood through the mitral valve causes the patient to have serious symptoms.

Less blood is ejected forward because the blood has two different directions to choose from; hence, the body does not receive its usual amount of fuel. This results in the feeling of fatigue and weakness.

Patients with regurgitation experience shortness of breath, because blood will back up in the lungs as noted in patients with mitral stenosis. Normally, blood flows smoothly from the lungs into the left atrium. But in patients with mitral regurgitation, some of the blood in the left ventricle returns to the left atrium, resulting in a buildup of pressure and a disruption of normal flow. Blood from the lungs now competes to enter the left atrium.

Drugs can help improve the symptoms of people who have mitral regurgitation. Unlike the case of narrowed valves in which the efficacy of drugs is very limited, medicines can improve matters with leaky valves. The amount of backflow of blood can be reduced with proper therapy.

Diuretics reduce the volume of fluid in the blood circulation. This, in turn, relieves some of the extra volume of blood in the heart. If there is less blood pumped by the heart, there is less blood to flow backward. Although this relieves some of the stress of congestion in the lungs, it is not the ideal way to treat the problem.

With diuretic use, there is less blood everywhere in the body because diuretics remove fluid indiscriminately. Although less blood builds up in the lungs (good), less is also ejected to the body (not good). The congestion in the lungs is treated at the expense of blood flow to the rest of the body.

Even so, diuretics are acceptable and at times even vital in the treatment of mitral regurgitation. But they are limited in their benefits, and clearly don't fix everything.

Vasodilators are an extremely important class of drugs for the treatment of mitral regurgitation. They act by dilating arteries and veins in the body, allowing for more blood to exit the heart, instead of flowing backward into the left atrium.

The ratio of blood flow (forward vs. backward) depends largely on the relative resistance that the blood has in each of the two directions. If the resistance to blood flow is reduced in one direction, more blood will flow in that direction.

Because they dilate the arteries of the body (making it easier to pump blood out of the heart), vasodilators lower the resistance of blood flow in the forward direction. More is pumped out of the heart, and less is pumped back into the atrium.

This is a more physiologic way to treat the problem than using diuretics. Vasodilators lessen the pressure in the lungs, while (in contrast to diuretics) improving the amount of blood flow to the rest of the body. Most patients with moderate to severe mitral regurgitation require *both* vasodilators and diuretics to relieve their symptoms.

Although drugs can improve the symptoms in most patients with mitral regurgitation, they do not fix the underlying problem. Drugs are temporizers, and eventually most of these patients need to have the valve replaced surgically.

Most people have surgery because their symptoms have become unmanageable despite medications. Surgery offers most of these people significant relief, but there are no guarantees. Some people do not improve dramatically, especially those with long-standing symptoms.

Others will develop serious and irreversible damage to their heart if the stress of mitral regurgitation is not eliminated. Fortunately, this does not happen to everyone, but we can't predict with certainty who these people will be. This is a difficult decision in clinical cardiology.

We are currently refining our ability to predict which patients should have surgery to protect their heart, even if they feel relatively well. Large scientific studies are in progress to observe who does well, and who does poorly, and when to operate. Waiting too long to operate on the high-risk patients can be a serious mistake. It is possible to pass the point of no return. These patients will not get better, even after open-heart surgery, once severe damage is done.

AORTIC REGURGITATION

When the left ventricle squeezes blood out of the heart, it exits through the aortic valve. After beating, the heart relaxes and begins to fill up with more blood. During this period of time, the aortic valve closes, so that the blood which has already been ejected out of the heart continues to move forward. The heart does not want that blood to return into the left ventricle after it has been ejected into the aorta.

However, in patients with aortic regurgitation this backflow occurs. Although most of the blood travels forward through the aorta to supply the body with fuel, some of it travels backward into the heart. This causes a characteristic high-pitched murmur during diastole. But, as with mitral regurgitation, there are physical findings that go well beyond the heart murmur.

To a greater degree than with mitral regurgitation, the backflow of blood in aortic regurgitation robs the body of the flow of blood. Much of the blood returns to the heart before it can reach its intended destination, resulting in serious fatigue, weakness, and problems with other organs of the body.

Since all organs receive their supply of blood from the heart, they all suffer when the net amount of blood that is ejected forward is reduced. The heart itself can suffer, resulting in chest pain during physical activity.

Additionally, the heart suffers from a backup of blood, similar to the situation in mitral regurgitation. The extra volume of blood that returns into the left ventricle causes pressure to build up in that chamber. This pressure is transmitted into the left atrium and the lungs, and results in congestion of blood in the lungs, which in turn produces shortness of breath with physical activity.

As with mitral regurgitation, drugs can help reduce the

symptoms of aortic regurgitation. Diuretics and vasodilators are helpful for the same reasons that they improve matters in mitral regurgitation. And, likewise, surgery is required in some patients to improve symptoms. In other patients surgery is required to prevent irreversible changes in the heart once the stress of the illness begins to take its toll. The management issues of aortic regurgitation are very similar to those of mitral regurgitation.

Mitral Valve Prolapse

Myth #5:
Mitral valve prolapse is a serious condition. Having mitral valve prolapse is always bad.

There is probably no cardiac diagnosis more overrated by the public than mitral valve prolapse (MVP). It is an inherited abnormality of the mitral valve of the heart that may affect up to 7 percent of all adults (an estimated 15 million Americans).

There are many fears about this condition. Most are totally groundless. Uncommon reports of strokes, arrhythmias, and sudden death among people with mitral valve prolapse have contributed to the exaggerated public concern.

These reports must be put into perspective. Mitral valve prolapse is not a simple, single condition. There are many different degrees of prolapse, some of which are more serious than others. But the overwhelming majority of people with MVP are totally healthy.

A very small number, on the other hand, have a more serious variant. These people can have mild to severe mitral valve regurgitation associated with their MVP, and may even require surgical valve replacement. Unfortunately, the prognosis of a healthy person with MVP is often confused with that of the more serious variants.

Sandy H. is a thirty-five-year-old woman with mitral valve prolapse. She was not aware of it until her doctor informed her that she had the condition three years earlier. Sandy had never had any symptoms or medical problems.

However, her life-insurance carrier increased her premiums after it was informed of the mitral valve prolapse. "You have a heart condition," the carrier stated, "and you could die from it."

This is a completely false conclusion. Sandy is healthy and has a normal life expectancy. Although anyone can die suddenly, Sandy is not at an increased risk because of her mitral valve prolapse.

Sandy fought her insurance company. Her cardiologist submitted a written summary of the implications (actually, the *lack* of implications) of her MVP, and the company lowered her rate to her previous level.

Some insurance companies are ignorant (or intentionally exploiting the hysteria) of mitral valve prolapse. Once an abnormality of any magnitude is discovered in the heart, people usually assume the worst. This creates undeserved anxiety. It is simple misinformation.

Some patients actually become sicker after being told they have mitral valve prolapse. If they have either vague chest pain or palpitations (feeling the heart beat quickly or strongly), they commonly have a worsening of their symptoms after learning their diagnosis. This is very likely to be related to the anxiety of being told of heart disease.

Myth #6:
"Having mitral valve prolapse means I will have
a heart attack."

The risk of having a heart attack is no different in people with mitral valve prolapse than it is in those with normal mitral valves. Heart attacks are caused by obstructions in the arteries running on the surface of the heart. The mitral valve does not contribute to this problem.

Mitral valve prolapse, on the other hand, does not protect from heart attacks either. People both with and without MVP can have heart attacks and sudden death for other reasons. Those with MVP are considered at the same overall risk as those without it.

Much of the poor comprehension of mitral valve prolapse results from a basic misunderstanding of what is actually wrong with the mitral valve. What is prolapse?

This is easiest to understand if we again compare the mitral valve to swinging saloon doors. The mitral valve is normally made up of two leaflets that work like the saloon doors.

Imagine what would happen if the saloon doors were built with the wrong materials. Assume that soft, flexible material was chosen instead of that which is usually firm and hard. Also assume that one of the doors was built with too much material, making it too long.

In contrast to the normal doors, which shut firmly, these saloon doors buckle when they close. The soft, extra-long door will bend when pressure is put on it.

This is essentially what occurs in mitral valve prolapse. In these patients the mitral valve is constructed of a somewhat floppy material. What's more, one of the leaflets is too long. Thus, the valve buckles easily when it closes. The extra length of the valve makes it more likely to buckle. The valve buckles

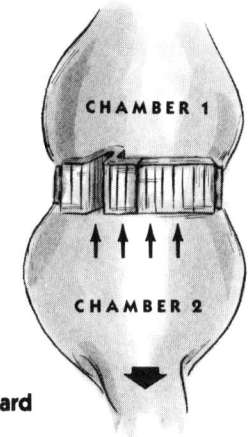

**Mitral valve prolapse:
Saloon doors buckle backward**

back into the left atrium because the pressure on the valve comes from inside the left ventricle. Hence, we say the mitral valve prolapses backward.

When the valve buckles, it causes a click, which can be heard with a stethoscope. But some people with MVP have more than the click of the buckling valve; they have a murmur of mitral regurgitation as well.

In these patients, the valve is extremely soft and floppy. When their valve shuts closed, under the pressure generated from the left ventricle, the leaflets do more than buckle. They actually swing backward into the left atrium, causing mitral regurgitation. This can vary from mild to severe regurgitation, but it certainly can be the most serious consequence of mitral valve prolapse.

It is estimated that from 10 percent to 15 percent of patients with mitral valve prolapse have some degree of mitral regurgitation. However, only a minority of these patients will eventually require surgery for severe symptoms. The remainder have a murmur, but with either no symptoms or only mild symptoms.

There are some symptoms that are classically related to mitral valve prolapse. They are considered part of a syndrome because of their common affiliation with MVP, although most of them are totally harmless. These symptoms include: anxiety (which often worsens after being told of the prolapse), chest pain, shortness of breath, palpitations, and fainting. Up to 50 percent of patients with MVP have one or more of these symptoms. Some patients with mitral valve prolapse have documented arrhythmias, which require drug therapy for suppression.

A small number of patients will develop an infection of the mitral valve. Any infection of a valve of the heart is called endocarditis, which is a very serious problem. Fortunately, this will affect fewer than 1 in 2,000 patients with mitral valve prolapse every year.

Any abnormality of any heart valve will change the flow of blood around that valve, causing little turbulences. These turbulences increase the likelihood that bacteria will stick to the valves, causing an infection, and clots will form on the valve. The sicker the valve (with greater disruption of the flow of blood), the more commonly these complications occur. Antibiotics are sometimes recommended in patients with MVP for protection against infections. Aspirin is helpful in preventing clot formation.

Fortunately, stroke is extremely uncommon among the millions of patients with mitral valve prolapse. The majority of patients with mitral valve prolapse will remain asymptomatic and healthy all of their lives.

Myth #7:
*"If I have heart disease, I must take antibiotics before
I see my dentist."*

This is a common myth, found not only among the general
public, but shared by many dentists. Most patients with diseases of their heart valves will require protection with antibiotics before certain procedures. But most people with heart
disease (those having angina, heart attacks, and even following bypass surgery) do not require antibiotics.

> William L., a fifty-eight-year-old man, had a quadruple bypass
> operation. His dentist refused to perform a dental cleaning until
> William took antibiotics.

The dentist is wrong. William does not need to take antibiotics because of his bypass operation (although a recent
survey reported that 40 percent of dentists are unaware of
this[1]). Only *some* heart patients need to take antibiotics, and
only at certain times.

Antibiotics are given to patients in order to fight bacteria
which enter into the bloodstream. There are millions and
millions of bacteria in the mouth. Very aggressive dental
work, often associated with bleeding in the gums, pushes
some of these bacterial organisms into the patient's blood
circulation.

The body normally eliminates these bacteria, without any
difficulty, through its immune system. There are many parts
of the body including the lungs and spleen that "suck up"
bacteria floating in the blood, helping to prevent a serious
infection.

Those people with abnormalities of the valves (narrowed
and leaky) have turbulent blood flow in the heart. Normally

the smooth flow of blood rushes the bacteria right through the heart. But in patients with valvular problems the bacteria bounce around and have the opportunity to stick to the valve. This can turn into a disaster.

If bacteria have a chance to stick to valves in the heart, they can grow into a serious infection, called endocarditis. The body's immune system does not effectively reach the valves of the heart. Thus, the bacteria can safely flourish.

Antibiotics are given in order to kill the bacteria chemically before they stick to the heart. If taken prior to dental work, the antibiotics stay in the bloodstream and wait for the bacteria.

Besides aggressive dental work, medical procedures involving the urinary system and the digestive system can cause bacteria to enter the blood. Thus, these procedures require protection with antibiotics in patients with valvular disease.

Patients with surgically implanted artificial heart valves need the most protection. Artificial valves are almost a magnet for bacteria. Further, if bacteria stick to these valves, they are almost impossible to eliminate. Thus, those with heart-valve replacement often require intravenous antibiotics in large doses before dental work. This is done under a cardiologist's strict supervision.

Patients with narrowed (stenotic) and leaky (regurgitant) valves need serious protection as well. But they can often manage with less aggressive antibiotics than those with the artificial valves. Non-artificial valves do not attract bacteria as avidly.

Patients with mitral valve prolapse are encouraged to receive antibiotics before undergoing dental work. However, recent evidence suggests that prolapse alone does not require this protection. But those patients with prolapse *and* mitral valve regurgitation should take antibiotic prophylaxis.

Those patients with a flow murmur (without any valvular problem) do not need antibiotics. In fact, it has been predicted that if everyone with a flow murmur were given penicillin before going to the dentist, we would probably kill more people from penicillin allergies than we would save from endocarditis. Both events are very unlikely, but it is not worth it to treat indiscriminately all people with murmurs.

Those patients who have had heart attacks or bypass surgery do not have to take antibiotics—unless they also have abnormalities of the valves. But coronary artery disease alone does not place a person at high risk for bacterial infections.

Myth #8:
Surgically replacing a sick heart valve makes the heart
"as good as new."

This too is a commonly held belief. People want to believe that surgery can cure heart disease, but this is not the case. Heart-valve surgery certainly improves symptoms, and even saves lives (for some patients). But it is not a cure.

The muscle of the heart can become damaged under the chronic stress of heart-valve disease. In some cases the muscle can get stronger, but in many instances it does not. Some damage is permanent; thus, heart-valve surgery can't fix everything.

Even if the heart is strong, the artificial valves can create their own problems.

Sally P., a fifty-four-year-old woman, came to the emergency room because of severe shortness of breath. She was found to be in moderate congestive heart failure (water in her lungs), and was further discovered to have severe mitral valve prolapse, with associated severe mitral valve regurgitation. The leaky mitral valve was responsible for her shortness of breath.

After treatment with medications, Sally still noted shortness of breath with minimal physical activity (walking one block). An echocardiogram demonstrated that the heart was under significant stress from the leaky valve. There were clear signs of damage to the heart.

Surgery was recommended, and Sally underwent a replacement of her mitral valve (an artificial, metallic valve was put into her heart). She felt much better after the operation, and was soon able to perform activities previously too difficult to undertake.

Sally was sent home taking a powerful blood-thinning medication, called Warfarin (commercially known as Coumadin). All patients with metallic heart valves must take this medication for the rest of their lives because the metal strongly encourages the formation of blood clots.

Sally did well until five months after the surgery. She returned to the emergency room with a stroke. Despite the fact that she took Warfarin, her blood-thinning level had drifted back to normal, and she developed a blood clot. She survived the stroke, but remained paralyzed on the right side of her body.

The risk of stroke is just one of the potential problems with metallic heart valves. Warfarin, which is required to prevent clot formation and stroke, can *cause* serious bleeding, especially if the dose is too high. Bleeding throughout the body, including the brain, has been reported. Warfarin thus requires careful regulation to maintain the balance between taking too much (making bleeding more likely) and taking too little (increasing the chance of stroke). Fortunately, there is an alternative to replacement with a metallic valve and thus an alternative to warfarin therapy.

"Bioprosthetic" valves are heart valves taken from animals (usually pigs). They are natural and do not have a strong tendency to develop blood clots, although there is a very small chance of this occurring. As a result, blood-thinning medications are *not* required therapy for most of these patients.

These valves are not as durable as the mechanical valves. Up to 50 percent of the bioprosthetic valves will erode by ten years after the original operation, requiring a second operation to replace the bioprosthetic valve. The metallic valves are stronger and last longer. Some have survived for twenty-five years.

Therefore, there is a tradeoff between the two different types of heart-valve substitutes. The metallic valves have a greater chance of inducing clot formation and stroke; hence, the open-ended administration of Warfarin (a powerful blood thinner) is necessary. But, on average, they last longer than the bioprosthetic valves (not a minor point in someone who is young and does not want to face a second operation). With advancing technology, the newer bioprosthetic valves appear to be stronger than the older ones, but we do not have enough clinical experience yet to know their life expectancy.

Both the metal and bioprosthetic valves attract bacteria to stick to them, resulting in a high risk of infection. Infection of an artificial heart valve is a serious complication. Antibiotics have a difficult time eliminating the bacteria from an artificial valve (metal or bioprosthetic). More than 50 percent of these cases require surgery in order to clear the infection (by replacing the artificial valve with a new one).

〜〜〜〜

CHAPTER NINE

Heart Failure

Up to 1 percent of the United States population suffers from heart failure, a serious condition described by weakness of the heart muscle and the inability of the heart to perform its job adequately. Although a heart attack is often the cause of heart failure, surprisingly there are many other conditions that can be responsible.

Many people believe incorrectly that they have a weak heart because they experience shortness of breath, weakness, or fatigue. Even doctors can be misled by these symptoms, and some patients are inappropriately prescribed cardiac medications when the problem is not with the heart.

Myth #1:
"If my heart muscle is weak, then I've had a heart attack."

This is not true, as seen in the following example:

Lewis K., a fifty-three-year-old man, complained of worsening
fatigue and shortness of breath during physical activity. An
echocardiogram revealed that his heart muscle was profoundly
weakened, but a cardiac catheterization found his coronary arteries to be completely normal.

It was later discovered that Lewis consumed four to five ounces
of alcohol (vodka) each day, which was responsible for his heart
failure.

Although Lewis suffered from heart failure, he never had
had a heart attack. Although heart attack is the most common
cause of heart failure, it is not the only one. With Lewis,
alcohol was the culprit.

The death of heart muscle and subsequent heart failure,
not related to heart attack, is called cardiomyopathy, for
which there are many possible causes, including:

1. *Hypertension*. The heart muscle beats under increased
stress when the blood pressure is elevated, resulting in the
gradual weakening and ultimate death of that muscle in severe
cases. This can usually be prevented by control of the hypertension with medications.

2. *Alcohol*. Chronic excessive consumption of alcohol (as in
the case of Lewis) can be associated with the progressive
death of the heart muscle, resulting in congestive heart failure. Although the reason is not fully known, there is a pre-
sumed direct toxic effect of alcohol on the heart muscle. Once
diagnosed, complete abstinence is required. This may allow
the damage to reverse itself.

3. *Valvular Heart Disease*. Leaky heart valves and narrowed
heart valves both cause stress to the heart muscle and can

result in progressive damage. Although surgery is usually recommended before damage occurs, some patients suffer from irreversible muscle weakness before reaching medical attention.

4. *Viral*. There are a number of viral infections that can invade the heart muscle directly, resulting in weakness and death of the muscle, for which there is no known therapy. Some people will recover with minimal damage after the infection is gone, whereas others suffer from severe and irreversible cardiomyopathy and even death.

5. *Unknown (Idiopathic)*. When a cause cannot be identified for any given medical condition, we call it idiopathic. There is no therapy for cases of idiopathic cardiomyopathy, and the majority (75 percent) of patients die within five years of the onset of symptoms. In these patients we never know why their hearts had weakened.

Regardless of the cause, heart failure is a serious condition in which many symptoms (shortness of breath, weakness, and fatigue) manifest themselves. Heart failure is also responsible for a reduced life expectancy.

Myth #2:
"If I am short of breath, it is because my heart is weak."

Molly S., a seventy-nine-year-old woman who had once been a heavy cigarette smoker, complained of severe shortness of breath during physical activity. She could not climb a flight of stairs without stopping to catch her breath.

Her doctor heard what he assumed was fluid in her lungs with his stethoscope, told her she had heart failure, and prescribed a heart pill (called digoxin) and a water pill.

Because her symptoms did not subside, she underwent an echocardiogram, which demonstrated that her heart muscle was strong. Subsequently, a breathing test revealed that Molly had severe lung disease.

It is not always possible to determine by physical examination alone whether a patient's symptoms are caused by disease of the heart or lungs. Many patients are on cardiac medications (such as digoxin) without proper indication because their symptoms have been misdiagnosed.

The three major syndromes that must be distinguished are: 1. weak heart; 2. stiff heart; and 3. lung disease.

1. *Weak heart:* The heart has two main jobs to perform—it must eject blood forward with each beat to the rest of the body, and it must fill with blood before the next beat. When the muscle weakens, it has difficulty performing these tasks, resulting in characteristic symptoms.

A weakened heart will eject less blood than the amount demanded by the body, resulting in the symptoms of weakness and fatigue, which we call forward failure.

There are many other reasons for feeling fatigued besides heart failure (including anemia, a "sluggish" thyroid, a variety of chronic illnesses, and merely being "run-down" and "out of shape"). The presence of severe weakness and fatigue is not diagnostic of heart disease.

The medication digoxin works by pushing the heart muscle to beat stronger, and can thereby help patients with heart failure feel stronger. As discussed previously (page 194), vasodilators act by dilating the arteries of the body, thereby lowering the resistance of blood flow out of the heart. This helps the heart to beat stronger and allows for more blood to eject forward with each beat.

A weakened heart also has difficulty filling with blood in between beats. Difficulty with this vital function results in the buildup of blood in the circulation behind the heart as the blood waits to enter and fill the pumping chambers. This is called backward failure. Pressure inside the blood vessels subsequently increases, forcing fluid to squeeze out of the circulation and into the tissue of the body (called edema).

When this occurs in the lungs (where blood waits to enter the left side of the heart), the patient develops shortness of breath because the airways fill with water (called pulmonary edema or pulmonary congestion). A characteristic sound of air passing through this water, called crackles, can be heard with the stethoscope.

Blood can also build up in the arms and legs while waiting to enter the right side of the heart. Edema fluid is released in these locations. For patients with heart failure, it is more common to have swollen legs because gravity causes even more fluid to accumulate in the lower parts of the body.

Avoiding dietary salt helps to reduce the volume of fluid in the circulation. And diuretics also help to diminish edema by increasing the removal of fluid through the kidneys. Leg elevation, in taking advantage of gravity, also helps to clear excessive fluid.

The presence of edema does not automatically mean that there is heart failure. Varicose veins and poor circulation can be responsible, as well as hormonal changes. For example, women commonly get mild edema during their menstrual cycle. However, heart failure is always a possibility (until proven otherwise).

2. *Stiff heart:* This condition is *under*appreciated by doctors, and can be compared to blowing up a stiff balloon with air. It takes great effort to inflate it, but the air ejects normally when the balloon is released.

Likewise, a stiff heart beats strongly, ejecting adequate amounts of blood forward, yet fills slowly, causing blood to build up behind it. This can result in edema in the lungs, arms, and legs, without the associated forward failure seen in patients with weak hearts.

High blood pressure in its early stages is a common cause of a stiff heart. The walls will also stiffen if they fail to receive enough fuel. Hence patients with coronary artery disease, especially during heart attacks, frequently develop this problem.

Edith M., a fifty-two-year-old woman with high blood pressure, complained of shortness of breath whenever she walked quickly. She was treated as if she had a weak heart with digoxin and water pills, but her symptom persisted.

Her breathing test was normal. The heart was found to beat strongly on an echocardiogram, and she had a normal stress test. Edith underwent a cardiac catheterization, which revealed normal coronary arteries. But the test also showed that the pressure of fluid inside of her lungs was significantly elevated.

Edith had a stiff heart, resulting in the elevation of pressure and the buildup of fluid in her lungs, causing her to experience shortness of breath. It is easy to measure the strength of the heart muscle (the echocardiogram actually visualizes the contraction), but it is more difficult to appreciate the stiffness of the walls. A cardiac catheterization is often required to measure the pressure inside the heart and lungs confirming the buildup of fluid.

Digoxin, which strengthens the heartbeat, is not a useful drug in these patients. It did *not* help Edith. The heart is not too weak, but too stiff. In fact, the ideal medications are those that actually cause the heart muscle to weaken slightly, and thereby relax, allowing for the normal filling of blood.

There are two classes of such drugs in common use: beta-blockers and calcium-channel blockers. These drugs may be dangerous in patients with weak hearts because they worsen the forward failure, but they are helpful in patients with strong, yet stiff hearts.

3. *Lung disease:* Patients with lung disease can experience many of the same symptoms as those with either weak or stiff hearts. Crackles can be heard in these respiratory patients, but the sound is caused by air traveling through collapsed airways, and not by traveling through water, as in heart failure. It is difficult to tell by listening with a stethoscope whether crackles come from disease of the heart or the lungs.

When a patient complains of shortness of breath, weakness, or fatigue, it becomes important to consider all the previously named conditions. By evaluating the lungs (with breathing tests) and the heart (by an echocardiogram, and an exercise test), most conditions can be properly identified and treated. In the more complex cases, cardiac catheterization may be required to establish the diagnosis.

Many patients are treated without the benefit of a complete evaluation. Some are on heart drugs, when the real problem is in the lungs. And some are on drugs (like digoxin) to strengthen the heart, while their problem is that of a stiff heart.

Myth #3:
Medications can make a weak heart strong again.

Although medications (like digoxin and vasodilators) can, while administered, improve the strength of the heartbeat, they can't reverse the underlying disease of the muscle. Muscle damage is generally irreversible, although there are occasional examples in which the muscle improves spontaneously.

Vasodilators have been demonstrated to improve the life expectancy of patients with heart failure. For example, one scientific study demonstrated that 52 percent of patients who took a placebo died during the one year they were observed, whereas 36 percent died during the same interval while taking a vasodilator (called enalapril).[1] Although this is a big improvement, mortality remains very high, even with medications.

Digoxin and water pills can improve the symptoms of heart failure, but neither has been demonstrated to have any impact on survival. Water pills must be used with caution, because they can deplete the body of potassium (an important mineral), and thereby make the body vulnerable to dangerous changes in the electrical rhythm.

Steroids were once thought to be helpful therapy for patients with cardiomyopathy. However, recent studies have demonstrated that they have minimal benefit and, in the doses required, have serious side effects.

For patients with severe cardiomyopathy, medications may fail to make a meaningful difference. In these cases, cardiac transplantation must be considered.

Valerie L., a twenty-eight-year-old woman, developed severe shortness of breath after delivering her first child. She was found to be in pulmonary edema (water in the lungs), and her heart was found to be profoundly weakened (the ejection fraction was 15 percent).

Medications (vasodilators and diuretics) helped to remove fluid from her lungs and improve her breathing, but Valerie still found her life to be very limited. She was unable to care for her baby because of her weakness and easy fatigability, and she became short of breath with minimal physical activity. After two months, without improvement, she was referred for cardiac transplantation.

This is a very sad case. Although its occurrence is very rare, some women (like Valerie) will, for unknown reasons, develop a cardiomyopathy after childbirth. Besides being severely limited by symptoms, Valerie also has a very poor prognosis (up to a 50 percent chance of dying within the next year). Cardiac transplantation is her best alternative.

Myth #4:
Cardiac transplantation is experimental, and probably won't work.

This is a common perception of cardiac transplantation, but it is untrue. It is hardly experimental, with more than 1,000 such operations performed each year in the United States (from more than 70 active transplantation programs). And the rate of survival is better than most people appreciate.

Although only 20 percent of patients survived for five years when the procedure was first introduced (in 1967), we currently see 80 percent survive the first year, and more than 60 percent survive for five years. The longest survivor, to date, has been healthy for more than eighteen years after his heart transplantation. The use of a drug called cyclosporine is mainly responsible for the improved survival statistics.

The biggest barrier to transplantation is rejection; the patient's body identifies the donor heart as foreign, and makes antibodies to attack it. Cyclosporine inhibits the body's immune system, and improves the chance of accepting the donor heart. But it also makes the patient more vulnerable to major and life-threatening infections. Close surveillance is required at two- to four-week intervals after surgery to look for both infection and rejection in these patients.

There are approximately 15,000 suitable candidates each year for heart transplantation. However, the number of donor hearts that become available ranges between 1,000 and 2,000 a year, forcing transplantation centers to select only the most suitable patients while rejecting the majority of the others. Priority is given to younger, and otherwise healthier, patients who have the best chance for success.

/\/\/\/\/\/

CHAPTER TEN

Personality, Exercise, and Alcohol

Certain risk factors have been clearly demonstrated to increase the likelihood of developing heart disease: cigarette smoking, diabetes, high blood pressure, and the presence of heart disease in closely related family members. However, there are other factors that have a more vague influence on the heart, including personality, exercise, and alcohol. There are many myths concerning what is proven about their relationship with the heart.

Personality and Stress

Myth #1:
People with "type A" personalities are the ones who die of heart attacks. Those with "type B" personalities are protected.

Although personality may influence the heart, this statement is exaggerated.

Since the mid-1950s there has been great interest shown by both the scientific community and the public in the effect of personality on one's health. There is a widely held perception that people with aggressive and hard-driven personalities are destined to have heart attacks, while those who are more relaxed are protected. This has not been scientifically established.

Personalities have been conveniently divided into two basic types (A and B) by psychologists. A type-A personality is defined by a strong sense of time pressure, an inability to relax, easily aroused hostility and aggression, and an extreme dedication to achievement. Type-B personality is one that is more relaxed and is defined by the lack of the previously mentioned type-A qualities. Those with type A have been commonly called "hyper," while those with type B have been labeled "mellow."

Scott B., a sixty-two-year-old corporate vice-president, had a heart attack during a business meeting. He was an extremely hard-working, aggressive, and demanding executive who had little patience for slowness and inefficiency.

During his ten-day hospitalization, Scott insisted on calling his office once or twice a day. Although he was advised to stay home and take it easy for six weeks after his discharge from the hospital, he returned to work in three weeks. "I feel well. It's silly for me to sit at home!"

Scott's friends were not surprised that he had a heart attack. "He has always been a pressure cooker. This was bound to happen," said one.

Here is a classic case that suggests to many people that Scott had a heart attack because he was so aggressive. It is easy to remember *his* heart attack and to blame his aggressive personality. Scott's friends believe that if he had a more relaxed personality, he would be in better health.

This is not necessarily true.

Jay P., a sixty-one-year-old barber, had a heart attack while watching television. Because he was a relaxed and easygoing person, his wife was surprised. "He is the last person who should have had a heart attack."

Even relaxed people with type-B personalities have heart attacks. Being relaxed does not offer immunity to heart disease, nor does having a type-A personality guarantee it. The current controversy debates whether those with type-A personalities are statistically more likely to have heart attacks than those with type-B. Is there a cardiac-prone personality?

The medical community is divided on this issue. Initial scientific studies performed in the 1950s and 1960s suggested that those with type-A personalities *did* have more heart attacks. These results were highly publicized, and were responsible for the public's exaggerated perspective on personality.

The most important of these studies, called the Western Collaborative Group Study, followed more than 3,000 men throughout the 1960s.[1] Those with type-A personalities had more deaths than those with type-B personalities. Although the difference was statistically important, it translated to only 16 extra deaths for every 1,000 people who were type A every decade. This is not an extremely large number.

Several less important studies published during the early 1970s also suggested that a type-A personality was cardiac-prone. However, more recent studies have been unable to demonstrate an increased incidence of heart disease among people with type-A behavior. The issue is, at best, murky.

In fact, in 1988 a scientific paper suggested that it might even be beneficial to have a type-A personality.[2] Among patients who had heart attacks, those who were type A had fewer deaths after hospital discharge than those who were type B. It has been hypothesized that type-A patients are more driven and motivated to monitor their symptoms, take their medications, and to quit smoking. Type-A behavior, therefore, may at times be protective.

With the conflicting information available in the medical literature, type-A behavior can't be considered to be an established risk factor for premature heart attacks and cardiac death.

Probably it has been too simplistic to divide personalities into only two types (A and B) in the first place. There are many variables that make up the human personality and therefore two basic types can't account for all these differences. With a better understanding of personality, it may be possible to describe some more specific types that are truly more susceptible to heart disease.

Recent scientific efforts have focused on a specific subgroup of people with a type-A personality: those with the most aggressive and hostile personalities. These people may be the ones who have a greater tendency toward developing heart disease.

But even if this is so, it will only reflect an increase in the statistical likelihood of developing heart disease. No type of personality will ensure premature illness. And certainly no personality type, even the most relaxed type-B individuals, can be guaranteed safety.

Therefore, the commonly held belief that type A is all bad and type B is all good is oversimplified and incorrect. Future research may help answer some of our questions about the influence of personality on the heart, but for now we have limited data that are, at best, conflicting.

Myth #2:
People with heart disease will die when they are emotionally upset.

We see movies in which someone dies of a heart attack after having an argument. But this is not when most heart attacks occur.

Only 15 percent to 20 percent of all sudden deaths and heart attacks occur after an identifiable event to which blame can be attributed, such as intense physical, emotional, or mental activity. The majority (80 percent to 85 percent) occur during sleep or restful activity.

During a moment of emotional stress the chance of having a heart attack is increased, but only by a small amount. And the amount of time spent during stressful moments is not long compared to the total time spent sleeping or resting. Hence, stress cannot be blamed for most cardiac events.

Exercise

During the past two decades there has been an explosive public interest in exercise. While only 126 people ran in the New York City Marathon in 1970, more than 20,000 participated in 1989. Health clubs have opened in many communities, and exercise videotapes have brought training programs into the home.

Besides the desire to feel better, many people participate with the hope of improving their life expectancy. In contrast, others remain inactive, fearing the dangers of intense activity. But, regardless of their perspective, most people have misunderstood the risks, benefits, and promise of exercise.

Myth #3:
If you exercise, you will live longer.

Most people who exercise regularly want to believe this is true. However, the scientific studies performed to date have not convincingly demonstrated that physical activity results in an improved survival rate. There is no proof.

A major investigation, from Harvard University, examined the level of physical activity of 16,936 college graduates, aged thirty-five to seventy-four.[3] The study, which examined the health of these alumni, found that those who exercised regularly lived longer than those who did not. But there are two problems with this study—the improvement is not as large as many had hoped, and the design of the study is flawed.

The study predicts that if a man (aged thirty-five to forty) exercises regularly, he will, on average, live an extra two to two and one-half years beyond what would be expected if he were inactive. Of note, this man would have to spend a cumulative time of more than one year exercising in order to live the extra two years.

The Harvard study had a significant flaw built into its design—it compared people who chose to exercise to those who *chose not* to exercise. People are more likely to exercise if they feel well, and are healthier to begin with. In contrast, those who don't exercise will include more people with underlying health problems.

Therefore, the study demonstrates that people who choose to exercise will on average live slightly longer than those who do not choose to exercise. But this does not demonstrate that exercise is responsible for the improvement.

It would be more valuable to take a large group of patients and randomly assign half to an exercise training program, while the others remain inactive, eliminating the above-mentioned bias. A study of this nature would be extremely expensive and difficult to organize but it would be a more valid way to demonstrate the role of exercise.

Myth #4:
Exercise makes the heart stronger.

> Ray W., a seventy-two-year-old man who suffered a large heart attack, joined an exercise rehabilitation program several weeks after his hospital discharge. After two months in the program, Ray felt better and told his wife, "My heart is definitely stronger."

When patients participate in exercise training programs, they often assume that their heart becomes stronger. This is not the case. Physical training results in a sense of well-being because of other effects: 1. it improves the efficiency of the muscles of the arms and legs; 2. it improves the hormonal tone of the body, resulting in a lower blood pressure and heart rate; 3. it lowers the level of cholesterol; and 4. it improves the control of sugar in people with diabetes. However, exercise will not make the heart beat more strongly.

In fact, the reverse was demonstrated in a scientific study that examined men who joined an exercise program within fifteen weeks of experiencing a large heart attack.[4] The heart muscle actually became weaker in these men, perhaps indicating that the exercise was premature.

Myth #5:
Exercise is extremely dangerous.

We occasionally read in the newspapers about a teenaged athlete who dies during football practice, or a middle-aged man who collapses while jogging.

These examples are startling and they convince many people that exercise is very dangerous. However, this is an exaggerated concern. Although there is an increase in the risk of having a heart attack during exercise, it is not large. Further, it is increased only for the small amount of time spent engaged in the exercise.

Sudden cardiac death is very infrequent among young athletes. When it does occur the majority of victims are found to have abnormalities of the heart that had previously gone unrecognized. A good physical examination could have detected the majority of these problems. Regardless of a person's age, anyone who wants to engage in organized athletics should first have a complete medical checkup.

Most middle-aged men and women who die during exercise are smokers (greater than 70 percent), and most have severe blockages in the arteries of their heart.

In 1981, a forty-eight-year-old man from France died while running in the New York City Marathon (as of 1989, he represented the only death in the history of the race). The day was unusually hot (greater than 70° F.) and the man had been pushing himself beyond his usual limits. He was running his best time, according to a friend who accompanied him.

Although the Frenchman was a former smoker, he did not have a history of heart trouble, or any symptoms. However, the autopsy revealed severe blockages in all three of his coronary arteries.

This is not an uncommon finding. Severe blockages can develop in the arteries of the heart without the knowledge of the patient. Therefore, most middle-aged people should have a stress test before engaging in an exercise program (in order to screen for serious heart disease). It is probable that the French marathon runner would have discovered through such a test that he had heart disease and may not have run that day.

Myth #6:
A stress test is very dangerous.

A patient once summarized her fear by stating: "I don't understand why they have to put me through stress to find out if I have trouble with my heart."

In reality, the stress test is very safe. A recent review (of more than 71,000 tests) found that the overall cardiac complication rate was lower than 0.8 (heart attacks or deaths) per 10,000 people studied.[5] The overwhelming majority of people had no problems.

A stress test is merely a means of observing the performance of the heart with an electrocardiogram during a period of gradually increasing levels of physical activity. It is also called an exercise test. There is no extraordinary stress involved.

A normal heart will perform normally on such a test. If there are blockages in the coronary arteries the test will usually indicate that there is a problem. But even for patients with heart disease, the test is safer than performing the same activity at home, because it occurs under medical supervision.

Alcohol

Myth #7:
Alcohol is good for the heart. / Alcohol is bad for the heart.

These opposing statements summarize the public's perception of alcohol: some people state emphatically that alcohol is toxic, while others argue that it is a tonic. In reality, alcohol has no significant cardiovascular effect on the majority of people who drink.

Alcoholic beverages have been consumed throughout the history of humanity. Yet, in relatively recent times, the dangers of alcohol consumption have been recognized and greatly debated.

Currently 10 percent of American adults are heavy users. In large urban areas, liver disease (from alcohol) is the second most common cause of death among people aged twenty-five to forty-four years old. Alcohol is responsible for the majority of fatal car accidents. And the emotional impact of alcoholism (on entire families) has recently been acknowledged to be widespread.

Yet, certain scientists have claimed that there are good effects of alcohol on the heart (especially when used in moderation). Several large-scale studies have demonstrated that people who consume, on average, from 0.5 ounces to 2.2 ounces of alcohol every day have slightly less heart disease than teetotalers.[6] And other studies have reported that alcohol consumption will increase (as much as exercise will, according to one investigator) the levels of "good" cholesterol in the blood.

In contrast to these benefits, alcohol is toxic to all cells in the body, including the heart muscle. Although alcoholic liver disease (called cirrhosis) is well known to the public, there is a less-known heart condition that is associated with drinking: alcoholic cardiomyopathy (cardiomyopathy is any weakening of the heart muscle).

This condition is characterized by severe weakness of the heart, resulting in general body weakness, shortness of breath, and the death of 50 percent to 80 percent of its victims within three years. It is believed to be caused by the direct "poisoning" of the cells of the heart by alcohol. We do not understand why this devastating condition affects only a small number of those who drink, but when it does occur, abstinence from alcohol is mandatory.

Alcohol can also provoke the heart to beat very quickly, causing certain arrhythmias to occur. This is seen during holiday seasons when more people tend to drink in excess, resulting in the term "holiday heart syndrome." Most of the arrhythmias will respond to abstinence and medications. Acute alcohol ingestion can be associated with sudden cardiac death but this is rare.

There is some truth to both of the original statements. Alcohol will certainly be harmful to a few patients by causing severe damage to the heart. In others, it will slightly lessen the likelihood of coronary artery disease. However, alcohol will have no significant cardiac effect in most. For those who do drink, it is better to drink in moderation (one or two ounces of hard liquor a day) than to consume greater amounts.

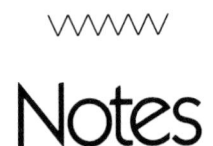

Notes

CHAPTER 1: CHOLESTEROL

1. The National Heart, Lung, and Blood Institute (a branch of the National Institute of Health) established cholesterol guidelines representing the U.S. government's official position (published in the *Journal of the American Medical Association*, 1985, p. 2080). The guidelines established were the result of a fourteen-person expert panel (entitled "The Consensus Development Conference on Lowering Cholesterol to Prevent Heart Disease") that examined evidence from dozens of medical studies, and interviewed twenty-two cholesterol experts, in 1984.

2. The graph is based on information supplied from "The Framingham Study: An Epidemiological Investigation of Cardiovascular Disease: the Eighteen-Year Follow-Up," Washington, D.C., Department of Health, Education, and Welfare, Publication No. (NIH) 74-599, 1974.

3. "The Lipid Research Clinic's Coronary Primary Prevention Trial" (LRC-CPPT) was published in the *Journal of the American Medical Association*, 1984, p. 351. The study was organized by the National Heart, Lung, and Blood Institute, and involved twelve participating lipid research clinics.

4. "The Helsinki Heart Study" (formally known as the "Primary-Prevention Trial in Middle-Aged Men with Dyslipidemia") was published in the *New England Journal of Medicine*, 1987, p. 1237. This study was organized by the University of Helsinki, and involved thirty-seven clinics throughout Finland.

5. "A Co-Operative Trial in the Primary Prevention of Ischaemic Heart Disease using Clofibrate" was published in the *British Heart Journal*, 1978, p. 1069. More than 15,000 men were enrolled (and clinically observed for more than five years) from three European medical centers, located in Edinburgh, Budapest, and Prague.

6. The American Heart Association published its cholesterol guidelines, entitled "Diet and Coronary Heart Disease," in *Circulation*, 1978, pp. 762A–766A.

7. The "Committee on Nutrition" of the American Academy of Pediatrics published its guidelines, "Toward a Prudent Diet for Children," in *Pediatrics*, 1983, pp. 78–80.

8. The "Food and Nutrition Board," Division of Biological Sciences of the National Research Council, published its results, entitled "Guidelines Toward Healthful Diets," in the *National Academy of Sciences*, 1980, pp. 8–12.

9. "Dietary and Pharmacologic Therapy for the Lipid Risk Factors," published in the *Journal of the American Medical Association*, 1983, pp. 1873–97.

CHAPTER 2: HYPERTENSION

1. "Comparison of the Effects of Diuretic Therapy and Low Sodium Intake on Isolated Systolic Hypertension," published in the *American Journal of Medicine*, 1984, pp. 1061–66.

2. The information in the table has been extracted from several scientific studies performed during the past three decades, including: 1. "Veterans Administration Cooperative Study Group on Anti-Hypertensive Agents: Effects of treatment on morbidity in hypertension. I. Results in patients with diastolic blood pressures averaging 115 through 129 mm Hg," in the *Journal of the American Medical Association*, 1967, pp. 1028–34; 2. "Veterans Administration Cooperative Study Group on Anti-Hypertensive Agents: Effects of treatment on morbidity in hypertension. II. Results in patients with diastolic blood pressures averaging 90 through 115 mm Hg," in the *Journal of the American Medical Association*, 1970, pp. 1143–52; 3. "Australian Therapeutic Trial in Mild Hypertension," in *Lancet*, 1980, pages 1261–67; and 4. "Medical Research Council Working Party: Medical Research Council trial of treatment of mild hypertension: Principal results," in the *British Medical Journal*, 1985, pp. 97–104.

3. "Primary Prevention with Metoprolol in Patients with Hypertension," in the *Journal of the American Medical Association*, 1988, pp. 1976–82.

CHAPTER 3: BYPASS SURGERY

1. "Coronary Artery Surgery Study (CASS): A Randomized Trial of Coronary Artery Bypass Surgery," published in *Circulation*, 1983, pp. 939–50.

CHAPTER 4: ASPIRIN

1. "Protective Effects of Aspirin Against Acute Myocardial Infarction and Death in Men with Unstable Angina: Results of a Veterans Administration Cooperative Study," published in the *New England Journal of Medicine*, 1983, pp. 396–403.

2. These six trials are summarized in "Aspirin After Myocardial Infarction," published in *Lancet*, 1980, pages 1172–73, and in a review article in the *Israel Journal of Medical Science*, 1983, pp. 413–23.

3. "Randomized Trial of Intravenous Streptokinase, Oral Aspirin, Both, or Neither Among 17,187 Cases of Suspected Acute Myocardial Infarction: ISIS-2 (Second International Study of Infarct Survival) Collaborative Group," published in *Lancet*, 1988, pp. 349–60.

4. These studies are reviewed in an article, "Clinical Trials Evaluating Platelet-Modifying Drugs in Patients with Atherosclerotic Cardiovascular Disease and Thrombosis," published in *Circulation*, 1986, pp. 206–23.

5. "Preliminary Report: Findings from the Aspirin Component of the Ongoing Physicians' Health Study," published in the *New England Journal of Medicine*, 1988, pp. 262–64.

6. "A Randomized Trial of the Effects of Prophylactic Daily Aspirin Among Male British Doctors," published in the *British Medical Journal*, 1988, pp. 13–16.

CHAPTER 5: HEART ATTACKS

1. This information summarizes the clinical experience of The New York Hospital's Division of Cardiology, obtained by following the outcome of 1,200 patients from 1983 to 1986.

2. "Effectiveness of Intravenous Thrombolytic Treatment in Acute Myocardial Infarction," published in *Lancet*, 1986, pp. 397–402.

3. "Randomized Trial of Intravenous Streptokinase, Oral Aspirin, Both, or Neither Among 17,187 Cases of Suspected Acute Myocardial Infarction: ISIS-2," published in *Lancet*, 1988, pp. 349–60.

CHAPTER 6: SUDDEN DEATH

1. "Use of the Automatic External Defibrillator in the Management of Out-of-Hospital Cardiac Arrest," published in the *New England Journal of Medicine*, 1988, pp. 661–66.

CHAPTER 7: PALPITATIONS AND PACEMAKERS

1. "The Incidence of Unwarranted Implantation of Permanent Cardiac Pacemakers in a Large Medical Population," published in the *New England Journal of Medicine*, 1988, pp. 158–63, examined the indications for pacemaker implantation at thirty hospitals in Philadelphia County, between January 1 and June 30, 1983.

CHAPTER 8: HEART MURMURS

1. "Recommendations for Prevention of Bacterial Endocarditis: Compliance by Dental General Practitioners," published in *Circulation*, 1988, pp. 1316–18.

CHAPTER 9: HEART FAILURE

1. "Effects of Enalapril on Mortality in Severe Congestive Heart Failure: Results of the Cooperative North Scandinavian Enalapril Survival Study (CONSENSUS)," published in the *New England Journal of Medicine*, 1987, pp. 1429–35.

NOTES

CHAPTER 10: PERSONALITY, EXERCISE, AND ALCOHOL

1. "Coronary Heart Disease in the Western Collaborative Group Study: Final Follow-Up Experience of Eight and One-Half Years," published in the *Journal of the American Medical Association*, 1975, p. 872.

2. "Type-A Behavior and Mortality from Coronary Heart Disease," published in the *New England Journal of Medicine*, 1988, pp. 65–69.

3. "Physical Activity, All-Cause Mortality, and Longevity of College Alumni," published in the *New England Journal of Medicine*, 1986, pp. 605–13.

4. "Exercise Training After Anterior Q-Wave Myocardial Infarction: Importance of Regional Left Ventricular Function and Topography," published in the *Journal of the American College of Cardiology*, 1988, pp. 362–72.

5. "The Safety of Maximal Exercise Testing," published in *Circulation*, 1989, pp. 846–52.

6. A review of such studies appears in an article entitled "Alcohol and High-Density Lipoproteins," published in the *Canadian Medical Association Journal*, 1980, pp. 981–84.

234

Index

combination grafts used in, 63
as common operation, 55
cost of, 73
damaged heart muscle and, 68
double, 64
fatalities in, 73, 79
goals of, 56
heart attacks after, 71–72
heart attacks in, 68, 72
heart condition improved in, 67–68
internal mammary arteries used in,
    62–64
life expectancy after, 68
limitations of, 68–71
myths about, 57–65, 67–68, 71–82,
    83–85
narrowed arteries and, 69
procedure in, 61, 66–67
quadruple, 64–65, 67
recurring angina after, 81
risks of, 68, 73
saphenous vein grafts used in, 61–
    62, 63
second, 71
single, 64, 67
studies on, 73
sudden death and, 76
triple, 64
types of tubes used for, 61–64
unnecessary, 80–82
for unstable angina, 72

calcium-channel blockers, 213
calcium deposits, 106, 180, 183, 185,
    186
cardiac arrest, 133–34
cardiac catheterization, 56–59, 82
procedure in, 57
risks of, 57–58
for stiff hearts, 212–13
for valvuloplasty, 188
cardiac monitors, 155
cardiac risk factors, 10, 26, 32, 116,
    217–27
see also specific risk factors
cardiac rupture, 136–38
cardiac sonograms, see ECHO tests
cardiac transplantation, 214, 215–16
cardiomyopathy, 208–9, 214–15, 227
alcoholic, 227
cardio-pulmonary resuscitation (CPR),
    133–34, 135
AIDS and, 143
by bystanders, 142

defibrillation and, 141–42
by family members, 142
by fire fighters, 141
CASS (Coronary Artery Surgery Study),
    74–77
blockages and, 74
medical vs. surgical survival in, 74–
    76
operative mortality in, 74
survival data in, 74–75
on three-vessel patients, 75–77
catheterization, cardiac, see cardiac
    catheterization
catheters, atherectomy, 85
cellular debris, 106
chest pain:
causes of, 117
as mimic of heart attack, 117
valvular disease and, 179, 187
see also angina
chest wall muscles, 117
children:
aspirin for, 86–87, 100
heart murmurs in, 171
rheumatic fever in, 180–81
streptococcal throat infections in,
    181
valve abnormality in, 185–86
cholesterol, 1–26, 70, 106
arteries clogged by, 1, 4–5, 56
biological function of, 4, 5
definition of, 4
diet and, 2, 15, 16
effects of, 4–5
exercise and, 223
heart attacks and, 8
inherited, 5–6
levels of, in older vs. younger
    adults, 7
lowering of, 14–18
measuring of, 13
medication for, 2, 15–16, 17, 20,
    21, 22, 23, 26
myths about, 4–18
national levels of, 1–2, 24
normal levels of, 5–6
as public health issue, 1, 2, 7
risk of heart disease and, 5, 6
saturated fats and, 11
seeping of, 9
skin and tendon deposits of, 5
sticking of, 9
studies on, 2–3, 15–18
types of, 12–14

ventricular, *see* ventricular fibrillation
fish oils, 11, 78
flow murmurs, *see* functional murmurs
Food and Drug Administration (FDA), 49, 87, 126
Food and Nutrition Board of the National Academy of Science, 24–25
foods:
  cholesterol-free, 2, 12
  myths about, 11–12
  saturated fats in, 11–12
forward failure, 210, 213
fractionation, 14
functional murmurs (ejection murmurs; flow murmurs), 173, 174, 175, 186, 204, 205
  aortic stenosis vs., 186, 187
  in athletes, 174
  echocardiograms for, 175–76
  in pregnancy, 173, 175
  in thin people, 174
  see also heart murmurs

gallstones, 117
gastric upset, 117
  from aspirin, 93
gemfibrozil, 21
  accidental and violent deaths and, 22
GISSI (Gruppo Italiano Per Lo Studio Della Streptochinasi Nell'Infarto Miocardico), 127–29
Greenland, cholesterol levels in, 24

Harvard University, 98, 221
HCTZ (hydrochlorothiazide), 50, 51, 52
HDL (high-density lipoprotein), 12–14
headaches, 33, 88
health clubs, 221
heart:
  valves of, *see* valves
  ventricles of, 102–3
heart attacks, 2, 6, 101–31
  acute, 119
  angina vs., 118
  antibiotic for dental visits after, 202–4
  arterial condition before, 124–25
  aspirin after, 96–97
  aspirin for prevention of, 86
  aspirin while having, 97
  blockages during, 106–10

in bypass surgery, 68
cardiac risk factors and, 116
cardiac rupture after, 137
chest pain and, 117–18
chest pressure in, 115–16
counseling after, 123
definition of, 102
ejection fraction and, 112–15
electrical failure and, 139
electrocardiograms for, 118–19
emotional stress after, 123–24
exercise and, 221–25
heart failure and, 207
indigestion diagnosed as, 116
information on, 101
lack of oxygen and, 103
life-style modifications after, 133
low cholesterol and, 8
minimal plaque damage and, 120–121
mitral valve prolapse and, 199
multiple, 117
myths about, 115–25, 127–31
number of, 121–22
pain in, 116
personality and, 217–21
psychological impact of, 123
rapid defibrillation for, 140–42
salt and, 43–44
scientific studies on, 97
sexual activity after, 122–23
silent, 116
size of, 110–12
strength of heart and, 112–15
streptokinase for, 128
stress and, 221
stress tests and, 120–21
thinning of blood to prevent, 92–93
thrombolytic drugs and aspirin for, 129
see also ventricular fibrillation
heartbeat, *see* heart rate
heartburn, 116
heart failure, 207–16
  alcohol and, 208
  cardiac transplantation for, 214, 215–16
  causes of, 207–9
  lung disease and, 213
  medication for, 210, 214–15
  myths about, 209–16
  reduced life expectancy and, 209
  salt avoidance for, 45
  stiff hearts and, 210, 212–13